FIXING YOU™

BOOKS IN THE **FIXING YOU** SERIES:

Back Pain

Neck Pain & Headaches

Shoulder & Elbow Pain

Hip & Knee Pain

Foot & Ankle Pain

Back Pain During Pregnancy

FIXING YOU: ™

SHOULDER & ELBOW PAIN

SELF-TREATMENT FOR
ROTATOR CUFF STRAIN,
SHOULDER IMPINGEMENT,
TENNIS AND GOLFER'S ELBOW,
AND OTHER DIAGNOSES

RICK OLDERMAN
MSPT, CPT

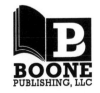

BOONE
PUBLISHING, LLC

2010 Boone Publishing, LLC

Boone Publishing, LLC

Editor: Lauren Manoy (lauren.manoy@gmail.com)
Interior Layout & Design: Lauren Manoy (lauren.manoy@gmail.com)
Medical Illustrations: Martin Huber (mdhuber@gmail.com)
Exercise Photographs: MaryLynn Gillaspie Photography

Boone Publishing, LLC
www.BoonePublishing.com

Library of Congress Control Number: 2009901653

Library of Congress Subject Heading:
1. Shoulder Pain—Physical Therapy—Treatment—Handbooks, manuals, etc. 2. Elbow Pain—Popular Works. 3. Shoulder—Care & Hygiene—Popular Works. 4. Elbow Pain—Exercise Therapy. 5. Self-care, Health—Handbooks, manuals, etc. 6. Shoulder Pain—Alternative Treatment. 7.Elbow Pain—Exercise Therapy. 8. Shoulder Pain—Prevention. I. Title: Fixing you: shoulder & elbow pain. II. Olderman, Rick. III. Title.

ISBN 978-0-9821937-3-0

Printed in the United States of America

Version 1.0

ACKNOWLEDGEMENTS

In science and medicine, we build on the shoulders of those who have discovered truths before us. Writing the Fixing You series has been no different. I would like to deeply thank Dr. Shirley A. Sahrmann for her breakthrough text, *Diagnosis and Treatment of Movement Impairment Syndromes,* on which the subject of this series is based. Were it not for her textbook and seminars, which I have immensely enjoyed, I would not have been able to write the Fixing You series, much less help so many people with chronic pain or injuries. Dr. Sahrmann is a rare breed of lecturer, therapist, and researcher with a sharp mind and wit to match. Her depth of knowledge in all things musculoskeletal and biomechanical leaves me speechless.

Additionally, I would like to thank Florence Kendall, Elizabeth McCreary, and Patricia Provance for their classic text, *Muscles: Testing and Function, with Posture and Pain.* This book has been a tectonic plate on which our understanding of orthopedic physical therapy stands.

THANK YOU!

I would like to thank Lauren Manoy for painstakingly editing this book. She has meticulously sifted through this information and helped me strike a balance between delivering technical information and making it digestible for you, my reader.

Thank you to Michelle for being my rehabilitation model as well as a star client!

Thank you Ken Margel and Scott Sturgis for shooting the rehabilitation video for me.

Thank you MaryLynn for the wonderful photos.

Thank you to Martin Huber for the illuminating medical illustrations.

Thank you to all my patients and clients who unwittingly served as my guinea pigs and those who wittingly modeled for pictures!

Last, thank you to my family for putting up with long hours of writing, meetings, and physical therapy speak.

This is dedicated to Russ.

CONTENTS

INTRODUCTION

Thirty spokes converge upon a single hub,
it is on the hole in the center that the use
of the cart hinges.

We make a vessel from a lump of clay,
it is the empty space within that vessel
that makes it useful.

We make doors and windows for a room,
but it is these empty spaces that make
the room livable.

Thus, while the tangible has advantages,
it is the intangible that makes it useful.

—LAO TZU

Fixing injuries requires, among other things, an understanding of anatomy and biomechanics. That is why this book and the others in my Fixing You series presents the Fixing You approach using clear and easy-to-follow language, case studies from my practice, and pictures and diagrams to guide you, the reader, in fixing your pain. My goal is to help you visualize exactly how your body works and what is going wrong when you experience pain. When you understand and can see clearly what causes your pain, you can develop and implement a plan to fix it using the exercises and tips outlined in the Fixing You series. But knowledge is only half the answer to the problem of chronic pain. True healing also requires adjusting your mental processes to work for you, not against you.

Attention to your body and how it is or isn't working is absolutely necessary to recover from chronic pain. In fact, lack of attention is a common factor in most peoples' health issues. Developing body awareness is often the most difficult—and most important—aspect of healing from chronic pain.

Intention is another intangible but crucial aspect of healing. Harnessing your intention—your singular focus toward getting better—will reap enormous dividends. Visualize it, verbalize it, write it down, and live as if you are getting better every day; in the process you will discover which habits are counter to your goals. Once you identify these habits, you can change them. Each change will reinforce your intention. The Fixing You series presents you with knowledge about the anatomy and biomechanics of injuries, and your attention and intention makes that information useful.

A NEW PERSPECTIVE

Since graduating from physical therapy school in 1996, I've spent hundreds of hours in continuing education classes and read countless professional journal articles and books that all attempted to answer these questions: Why do we have pain, and how do we fix it? I quickly realized there was more to injuries and healing than what I was taught in the courses I had been taking, although each had a piece of the puzzle. I realized that I needed a more complete understanding not only of how muscles and bones work, but how they work together to create movement.

Throughout my early years as a physical therapist, I tried one person's approach here and another's technique there. These various ideas about how to treat pain sometimes worked temporarily, but my clients didn't usually present or respond exactly like the case studies in the courses. Wanting to help people and not having the answers was frustrating. So I resolved to observe my patients closely, and I started to see the following patterns emerge:

- Patients resolving back pain using methods counter to traditional approaches.
- Chronic hamstring tightness and strains in athletes with strong hamstrings.
- Correcting structural issues in people with chronic neck pain and headaches only to have them return again and again.
- Knee pain in people whose leg muscles were strong and had good range of motion.
- Repeated straining of shoulder muscles in athletes whose musculature was strong.

In the meantime, I began exploring personal training over several years while working at an exclusive fitness club in Denver, Colorado. I had exercised all my life and found my work as a physical therapist limiting in terms of my career and life goals. Personal training seemed to be a natural extension of my interest in working with people within a larger spectrum.

My first client was a woman who was unable to raise her arm over her head. I reviewed her workout and found that she was doing all the wrong exercises for someone with her issues.

"Doesn't this workout hurt you?" I asked her.

"Of course it does," she replied. "Isn't it supposed to be painful?"

"No, it should be pain free," I said.

"What about 'no pain, no gain'?" she asked.

"No pain, no gain" is much like Nike's slogan, "Just Do It." You must understand that you still have to check yourself to be sure what you are doing is not harmful.

What may help one client may hurt another. I knew then that the fitness field needed more physical therapists. We are trained to not only assess joint and muscle function but to extrapolate that information into a performance model for sports, work, or just plain healthy living. Currently, the fitness industry includes personal trainers and Pilates, aerobic, and yoga instructors who are trying to help clients in pain but who have limited knowledge of anatomy or the optimal biomechanics of a healthy body—much less an injured one.

Working as a personal trainer gave me access to a type of injury that I hadn't much experience with: chronic pain. As a physical therapist in a sports and orthopedic clinic, the majority of my patients had acute injuries or surgical repairs. But there are thousands of people—if not millions—in the clubs and corporations across the United States who are exercising or working in pain, fighting chronic injuries that they've been dealing with for years, and trying to make themselves better. I know because I quickly became the busiest and highest-producing trainer/therapist at the club during my tenure there. At the time, and even now to a large extent, most people do not have access to physical therapists' musculoskeletal expertise. I was seen as something of a novelty. Thus began my quest to synthesize a more complete understanding of how dysfunction and injuries were related.

A BREAKTHROUGH

While treating one of my clients, I had an epiphany. Debbie had a 15-year history of neck pain and migraines after two back-to-back motor vehicle accidents, and she had tried everything and everyone to find relief. After a few sessions, I realized that her problem did not lie in her neck, but in her shoulder. I had made a critical connection that I hadn't thought about before: The structural damage the accidents had created wasn't the cause of her pain; it was caused by dysfunctional biomechanics that created vulnerabilities and which the accidents had exacerbated. We addressed these functional issues, and within a few days her pain had disappeared.

Just as I was finishing with Debbie, I discovered a book that confirmed my diagnosis and treatment approach with her as well as a few of my other chronic pain patients. Written by Dr. Shirley A. Sahrmann, a physical therapist out of Washington University in St. Louis, *Diagnosis and Treatment of Movement Impairment Syndromes* is a medical textbook that provided the missing links I had been seeking to pull together my observations. Many of the biomechanical paradigms and rehabilitative exercises in the Fixing You series have been adapted from Dr. Sahrmann's brilliant textbook. I recommend that all physical therapists purchase the book and attend her courses.

Another book I regularly reference is Florence Kendall, Elizabeth McCreary, and Patricia Provance's classic, *Muscles: Testing and Function, with Posture and Pain*. This textbook is a wealth of information for understanding precise musculoskeletal anatomy and testing. It is a standard in physical therapy, and I regularly refer to it for isolating muscle testing. It guides me in specifically analyzing and thinking creatively about function. By understanding muscle function on a basic level, I can better hypothesize functional deficits that may be occurring at a systemic level.

But my books are written for laypeople, not medical professionals, to guide you in healing yourself. I've simplified and distilled my medical training to reflect the majority of problems I've found when treating clients. I've prioritized the corrective exercises I've found most powerful for most conditions. I've bolded vocabulary words and added information boxes to help clarify words or concepts. I've also created videos of all the exercises and tests to enhance the effectiveness of your program. To view these free video clips, visit my website at **www.FixingYou.net**. Type in the code at the end of this book to access the extra material.

HOLISTIC FUNCTION

The body is the sum of individual units working together to create functional movement. Bones, muscles, tendons, nerves, and ligaments can all be addressed individually, but it is important to understand how these structures work collectively to fulfill a purpose: pain-free movement of the body. So, while it is imperative that individual "chinks in the armor" are found and corrected, visualizing how the whole works together is just as important. This concept also works from the other direction; training movement and/or function reinforces and assists in correcting the poor performance of individual muscles. In this book, I've introduced the key individual players—the parts that make up the whole—and also shown how they play together to create function, much like a symphony. You are responsible for bringing them in line to create your concert.

I wish you the best in your pursuit for solutions to your pain. You are not alone in your search for answers. I truly believe that, with a little thought and effort on your part, the Fixing You approach will help you find your answers, as it has for my clients.

The beauty of the body is that results happen quickly when you are doing the right thing. Most of the clients you will read about, and those that aren't included in this book, feel significantly better after only one or two treatments. Often, my clients understand they are on the right path within minutes of performing an exercise. Emboldened by this sense, they become more committed to the process of fixing themselves. You can have the same feeling of empowerment. There is no magical technique or device that will fix you. Only *you* can fix you—so let's get started on giving you the tools to do just that.

1 | MINDFUL HEALING

There is not a single problem in LIFE
you cannot RESOLVE, *provided you*
first solve it in your INNER WORLD,
its place of origin.

—PARAMAHANSA YOGANANDA

Time and time again I see clients who have tried so many unsuccessful cures that they just don't know what to do. This is worrisome—not because I believe I can't help them, but because they don't believe they can help themselves.

The most powerful aspect of the Fixing You approach is that it shows you what is wrong, actually getting you to feel that certain muscles or movements are not working and how your pain changes when they are corrected. This helps define the problem. It gives issues a beginning and an end, allowing you to compartmentalize pain and therefore see when and how the solution will happen.

Given the tools to understand and correct your injuries, I hope you will feel a sense of empowerment that will motivate you to work harder to fix yourself. If you can define an injury, then you have the power to fix it—and that motivation will get you results.

Getting your head into your plan is essential. Without your commitment, chances are it will never get done. The exercises and techniques I describe in this book will only help you if you commit to them—or more importantly, if you commit to yourself. You cannot pursue any program halfheartedly and expect to get the big payoff. If I find myself more committed than my client, our work is done. I cannot want it more than them. In my experience, there are three processes involved with positive change: You have to visualize the problem and the change needed to solve it, verbalize your intention and write down a plan of action to fix it, and take action to implement your plan.

Visualize the Problem

Visualization of ideal movement is difficult for many people with chronic pain conditions. This is largely because they are unfamiliar with the anatomy of their injuries or the reasons their injuries exist. The information in this book will help you "see" what's at the bottom of your pain and how to fix it by giving you a glimpse into the underlying anatomy.

You'll notice that as much as I discuss the anatomy of a problem, I also talk about movement. There's little use in learning anatomy if you don't also learn how it creates movement. You will learn what happens to your joints if your muscles are not working correctly and how that causes pain.

This brings me to another reason why visualization can be challenging. Most chronic pain is the result of years of poor movement habits—habits that have taken on the guise of "natural" movement, even though these are actually unnatural and harmful habits (also called **movement dysfunctions** or movement faults). For instance, you will discover that many people who experience shoulder or elbow pain have shoulder blades that don't move well. The shoulder blade is supposed to help the arm and forearm move. When it doesn't move well, the shoulder or elbow joints must then move more than they usually do. This excessive movement causes pain. Correcting these issues results in patients sensing they are using their arm in a different way—yet it feels better.

> Creating **positive change** involves internalizing your desire, verbalizing your intention, and acting on it.

This tells me that their sense of biomechanically correct movement is actually wrong. What they "visualize" as ideal movement needs to change. To this end, I often ask my clients to perform their exercises in front of a mirror to give feedback on their form. Most people have never taken the time to observe their movement patterns, and this is a real eye-opener for them.

Visualizing your shoulder blade's proper alignment will initially be a little awkward because it's located on your back and is difficult to check. But you'll quickly grasp this because you will soon learn that changing how you use your shoulder blade results in pain reduction. You will need to retrain your body's movement habits because chances are that you've been reinforcing your movement dysfunctions for years, if not decades.

In the case of muscles that aren't working correctly, visualize them scrunching up and getting shorter when trying to contract them, and visualize them lengthening when stretching. Tap the muscle briskly to get it to "wake up." As you will see by reading my clients' stories, healing a muscle that has been under chronic stress can occur almost instantly. The muscles only need to relearn how they should perform. In many cases, pain will instantly diminish or be eliminated altogether.

Look at the illustrations of key muscles in this book, and take some time to visualize where they are on your body and what they do. Using your fingers, feel the area in question to help yourself consciously connect with it. You may need a friend or spouse to actually put a hand on your shoulder blade while you raise your arm to develop your awareness of it and to help you see how it moves. Get a sense of where in the arm-raising movement it begins to move and stops moving. Developing this sense will be crucial to understanding the roots of your shoulder and elbow pain. Connect what their fingers are feeling to what your brain is experiencing. Then try it without touching your shoulder blade to see if you still get the connection.

> Set aside 10 seconds throughout the day to **get in touch** with your body and visualize its muscles.

Verbalize Your Intention

Solidify your ideas and support your intention to heal by talking to friends or family or writing down your plan. Often, discussing plans brings their fruition one step closer.

I think all of us have had a time in our lives where we secretly challenged ourselves to reach a goal but didn't tell anyone about it because saying it would heap more responsibility on our shoulders to make it come true. I've run into this situation countless times, where a client won't dare say they expect to become pain free for fear of not meeting their goal and being disappointed. Even when they become pain free, they still doubt that it will continue. Take the plunge and express your goal or desire to eliminate your pain. Put that responsibility on yourself. Hold yourself accountable for following through with this process of fixing your pain. Come up with a short phrase that affirms your intention, and repeat it throughout the day. "Every day, my body is working better and better" is an empowering statement that will help you keep a positive mental attitude. You can make this statement because it is completely realistic, as opposed to setting an unrealistic goal, like running a three-minute mile.

Your body is not designed to be in chronic pain. Something you are doing or not doing is perpetuating your condition. Commit to yourself by telling your friends and family about your goals. By telling friends and family that you believe you will become pain free, you have already made a shift in your consciousness to believe that it will happen. Say it! Your friends and family will probably offer to help you in any way possible. This would be a good time to ask them to put their hands on your shoulder blades while you move your arms!

So often in my life, when I'm working toward achieving a goal and getting hung up, I write about what I am doing and the problem I am facing. This small act helps me clarify what I need to do to get from point A to point B. Write down your thoughts and experiences in a journal. Track your progress. If you're getting stuck on a particular concept or exercise, write about it. What is it that you don't understand? Where are you getting stuck? The act of writing will help you see clearly where you are going wrong. It will also help you see what you are doing right and how far you've come since beginning to take action.

Write down how many hours (or minutes) of a particularly painful activity you can do before pain sets in. Write down how many repetitions of an exercise could be completed before you became fatigued. Check your progress in a couple weeks. Can you perform the activity longer before you feel pain? Can you do more repetitions before you experience fatigue? Have you learned a technique that eliminates your pain? Have you uncovered a habit that contributes to your pain?

All of these are great places to begin when tracking your progress. If you did something new that really hurt, then write it down. Figure out why it hurt. Make the necessary adjustments and see if those helped. On the other hand, if you found something that really helped, then write this down as well. It will be valuable information for you to implement later if you hit a plateau.

Physical therapists use **short- and long-term goals** to create our treatment plans—and you should do the same.

Create and write down two short-term goals like the following examples: "I will perform my exercises using correct form five times a day for the next week"; "I will set up 10 reminders at work, at home, and in the car to help me change my habits during the next week"; "In the next four days, I will identify 10 circumstances during which I notice my arms excessively rotate inward." Long-term goals should build on your short-term goals, like the following examples: "I will increase my exercise repetitions, using correct form, by 10 repetitions over the next four weeks," or "I will increase my exercise routine to include two strengthening exercises within three weeks."

Take Action to Implement Your Plan

Finally, you must take action to reach your goals. I guarantee that if you do not take action, your goals will not materialize. So often, I give clients exercises to practice that clearly are instrumental in fixing their pain. When I see them next, however, I frequently find they've only performed one or two sessions since our last visit. This is not the most effective way to address chronic pain.

When you have a chronic pain condition, one repetition of an exercise each day will not fix it. You may initially have to exercise several sessions each day until the length or strength of the involved muscles are at least partially corrected. Once this is accomplished, your pain will diminish, and you can begin whittling down the exercises.

Often, a maintenance plan is necessary because movement dysfunctions are what most likely got you into trouble in the first place. These will be more difficult to identify and correct because they are habits, and habits aren't easily broken. Throughout this book, I've offered some guidance for identifying common movement dysfunctions to help you recognize these and to get you started on correcting them. Ultimately, to permanently eliminate pain, these habits must be corrected.

Bringing your attention to what you are doing will be the most difficult aspect for many of you. In this book, you will find techniques and exercises to ease or eliminate your pain for good. You must, however, feel and notice how your body is moving and performing the exercises. Attending to your specific mechanics will deliver results. I see it all the time, and your body is built no differently than all the other people this approach has worked for.

With the demands of our busy days, it can be difficult to stay focused on these changes. That is why I recommend you set up a way to remind yourself of your new goals and to check in on your habits. Wear a special bracelet, ring, string, or rubber band around your wrist to remind you of the changes you are evoking in your mind and body. Place stickers on the dashboard of your car, the clock, your watch, your telephone—anything you use or look at frequently—to remind yourself that you are getting better every day by correcting those habits that feed your pain.

People often believe that they will have to permanently set aside a lot of time for exercise. Not true. I am asking you to make time over the next two to four weeks to heal yourself. If that doesn't sound realistic to you, then you need to rethink your priority of fixing yourself. Each session should take no longer than five to seven minutes, two to five times each day. In total, I am asking you to take 35 minutes a day for the next two to four weeks to get rid of years worth of pain. That doesn't sound too bad, does it?

THE MIND–BODY CONNECTION

A woman I treated during my first year out of physical therapy school is a great example of how powerful a tool the mind is in affecting our bodies. Iris was one of my first patients. Her diagnosis was intermittent cyanosis, which basically means that her extremities occasionally turned blue due to lack of oxygen.

Now, this isn't something we learn about in physical therapy school, so I took an extensive history that included a husband who had suffered a heart attack and been hospitalized a few months earlier. After this, Iris went home and scrubbed her house from top to bottom. The next morning she awoke with blue fingertips and lips. She went to see doctors, specialists, herbologists, acupuncturists—you name it. No one had a clue as to the solution, and neither did I.

I decided to do some range-of-motion and strength testing. As we began moving, her fingertips, toes, and lips turned blue. As a first year grad, I knew enough to know this wasn't good. So I gave her a few stretches, making sure she understood to stop if anything turned blue, and sent her home. After she left the office, I called the referring doctor.

"I just had Iris in here, and she turned blue during my exam," I began.

"Yes, we've seen that happen too," replied the doctor.

"Have you done blood tests to see whether there is a chemical cause for her symptoms since this seems to correlate to her cleaning episode?" I asked.

"We've run every test we can think of. Nothing abnormal shows up," replied the doctor.

"I've never seen this before," I said.

"Neither have we," said the doctor. "Just do your best. We have to exhaust all avenues, and she's been through just about everything and everyone."

After three days practicing stretches, Iris returned. "Still turning blue," she offered. She was visibly upset. In my mind, I believed there was no exercise I could offer her that would correct this problem. I went back to her history and we talked.

"Iris, your husband had a heart attack three months ago," I began. She nodded, looking concerned.

"How's he doing?"

"He's much better. He's just started a walking program." She brightened a little.

Then what I needed to say next came to me. I looked her straight in the eyes and said, "Iris, your husband isn't going to die." She blinked. "And neither are you," I continued. She blinked again and let out a deep breath.

I felt I was onto the source of her problem and continued, "Have you ever spoken of this to a therapist, counselor, priest, or friend? Anyone who you can confide in?"

"No, I haven't," she said.

"Then your treatment is to do so within the next four days. I'll see you in a week," I finished.

She came back next week, arm-in-arm with her husband and looking radiant.

"I just wanted my husband to meet you," she said and smiled. "This is him," she told her husband.

"How are you feeling?" I asked hopefully.

"No symptoms at all! Look!" She did all her exercises with no signs of cyanosis.

"Amazing," I said.

"I spoke with a therapist, and I feel so much better! I can do anything!" she exclaimed.

"Yes, you can," I said. We spoke some more and then hugged goodbye.

This has always struck me as a dramatic example of the mind's influence over the body. I cannot explain how her mind affected her blood flow the way it did, but the connection seemed clear. We read stories almost daily in the newspaper about similar phenomena—people holding on to their lives through sheer will after being trapped in an earthquake or becoming elite athletes after conquering a life-threatening illness. We've all read or heard about Eastern mystics able to control almost every aspect of their bodies through meditative practice. Tapping into your brain's power to control your muscles, monitor your habits, or feed your desire to become better will be a large part of you remaining pain free after identifying and fixing the physical issues causing your pain. If Iris can restrict blood flow to her extremities and then reverse it, then surely we can master the way we move and function, and thereby live pain free.

My experience tells me that no matter what diagnosis you have or what kind of accident you were in, the body must learn to move correctly in order for tissues be pain free or to experience significant pain reduction. This book teaches you to assess your movement patterns and correct the most common issues preventing ideal movement.

THE POWER OF WILLPOWER

Some people make goals because they'd like to achieve an end— and some people make goals because they *must* achieve an end. The second group are the people who get the work done, and usually above and beyond what I've asked of them. This is embodied in Ernie's truly inspirational story. Ernie had a traumatic brain injury as a result of being hit by a drunk driver while he was in a bike race. This happened three years earlier, and Ernie wanted to ride in that race again to prove to himself that he could do it. He had been through so much with his rehab, return to work, and family issues. This was one last big hurdle he wanted to clear.

I met Ernie and liked him immediately. I didn't have much experience working with people with brain injuries, just my clinical rotation during physical therapy school. I knew that these people need to limit stimuli (bright lights, loud noises, strength challenges, balance, and so on) because their brains have difficulty filtering the information.

But Ernie had fire in his eyes, and I could see he was committed in spite of his obvious challenges with cognitive, balance, strength, and flexibility deficits. We began by working in a dim, quiet room with no distractions and rigged up a bike with exercise stretch tubes to get him comfortable sitting on a bike again and relearning how to balance himself. I gave him instructions in simple sentences with plenty of time in between for processing. Once we mastered those skills, we moved on to standing balance and strengthening, while learning how Ernie's brain responded to physical exertion and simultaneously receiving instructions. He made excellent progress while we tailored his program to his specific needs.

I had the idea to make a set of training wheels for his transition to the bike outside. I visited several bike shops and spoke to their mechanics about my situation; each one told me to forget it, saying that I'd never get a person with a brain injury to ride a bike because it would be too difficult. That just fired me up even more. "You don't know Ernie," I thought.

Finally, we decided that I'd hold on to the bike while he rode. Ernie was scared at first, and so was I. If a person with a brain injury hits his head, he is more susceptible than the rest of us to further injury. Until that point it was relatively safe, innocuous work with no chance of further injuring his brain. But to achieve Ernie's goal of riding in his race, we had to take some risks. He had worked hard, and it was time to take the next big step.

Ernie and I went out to the parking garage, and he mounted the bike. I held on and ran with him while he pedaled and found his balance. We continued this for many sessions: I gave Ernie instructions, Ernie responded, and both of us learned how far we could push the envelope with this whole new level of difficulty.

Until one day Ernie said, "Let go."

"Are you sure?" I asked, huffing.

"Yes, I can do it. Let go," he answered.

I did. And he did.

He rode like a dream for 10 minutes. Once I saw his telltale signs of mental fatigue it was time to get off. While I held the bike for Ernie to dismount, I looked into his eyes. He was exhilarated and had engaged with plenty of stimuli for the day. Neither of us said a word. The hard work was done—then it was just a matter of building up his endurance.

I had never been as proud of someone as I was of Ernie that day in the garage. He stared down his fears and setbacks and rose above them in spite of all the evidence that he should not have been able to do what he did. He was and is a real hero and inspires me to this day. By the way, he rode in that race and finished, three years after being hit on his bike with only the chin strap of his helmet left intact. There is no reason you cannot achieve similar greatness and pride in your own accomplishments. You just have to begin.

Ernie faced his demons and conquered them. In spite of everything working against him, he drew from his vast inner strength to do what no one else believed he could do. Fixing chronic pain is no different, except with one caveat: Instead of others not believing in you, it is usually you who does not believe in yourself. It's no wonder, after seeing specialists and therapists who couldn't help you or after seeing images of structural damage and being told this was the cause of your pain. This time will be different because you will have the keys to unlock the mysteries of your pain.

Attention and Awareness

Chronic aches and pains aren't just for those who have been involved in accidents. I've found similar biomechanical problems at the roots of chronic pain in people who have had traumatic accidents as well as in those who didn't. Therefore, I believe accidents expose and exacerbate existing vulnerabilities in our bodies. Fixing someone who was involved in a motor vehicle accident that resulted in chronic back pain has been no different than helping someone who has had back pain for decades and has never been involved in an accident. They both require an understanding of how poor function is feeding the problem and what needs to be corrected to eliminate pain. Essentially, in order to fix your body and eliminate chronic pain, you need to pay attention to how your body moves.

I used to work at a health club. While I was in the locker room changing after a workout one day, a man approached me.

"Hey, do you mind taking a look at my arm? I bumped it last week, and now I don't seem to have the strength like I used to," he said.

"Sure," I said.

In three seconds, I knew exactly what his problem was; he had completely severed his biceps tendon at the elbow. His injured arm was visibly smaller than the other, and the biceps muscle was curled up in a little ball up by his shoulder, similar to the way blinds roll up on windows. It was as if someone had stuffed a sock into his upper arm.

"You've ruptured your biceps tendon," I said, "and you need to get an orthopedic surgeon to operate on it immediately."

He returned a few days later. "I saw a surgeon, and he said it wasn't torn," he said.

"Go see another surgeon—it's torn. I guarantee it," I said. "And do it fast!" I added.

I saw him a month later in the locker room. "You were right," he said. "I saw another surgeon, and I had an emergency operation that day."

This man was not in touch with his body. Many of you reading this book are in a similar situation—not ever considering how different parts of your body work together to create pain-free movement. In the above case, a man had suffered a traumatic blow to his arm that caused his problem. In this regard, it was a clear-cut issue that had an easily pinpointed cause. Chronic pain that isn't due to trauma is often caused by a gradual decline in the quality of the body's movements. It is time for you to pay attention to your body, and my sincerest hope is that the information in this book will help you do that. The exercises in this book will help you if you check in with yourself and become aware of your body. Always go back to your form and think about what you are doing. Be present and be attentive—you will be rewarded for it!

PAIN: THE GOOD AND THE BAD

The last item I'd like to address is pain avoidance. It is a natural reaction to avoid a stimulus that is hurting you. The operative premise here is that it is *hurting* you. Quite often I need to educate my clients regarding "good" pain versus "bad" pain. The discomfort of a fatigued muscle feels different than the pain of a muscle strain or **impinged** joint—pain that indicates injury. Learning to tell the difference between "good" pain (the temporary discomfort of retraining your body) and "bad" pain (pain that indicates injury) is important to your healing process.

Generally, what I'm referring to as "good" pain is a feeling of fatigue in the muscles or tissues you are exercising or trying to restore range of motion to. Muscle fatigue may be uncomfortable, but it doesn't mean that what we're doing is hurting us—in fact, that feeling of fatigue lets us know that we are getting stronger. Muscle fatigue also indicates that your body has had enough for the time being. Listen to your body. Stop when you need to. Don't try to push through another set of repetitions or add more weight until your body is ready. Avoiding the message your body is sending doesn't do you any favors and ultimately slows down your progress because ignoring good pain establishes compensatory behavior that can contribute to bad pain.

> **Slow down** and feel what your body is telling you when performing the tests and corrective exercises and when you're out and about during the day.

For example, imagine that you are performing a biceps curl, bending your elbow to bring your hand to the top of your shoulder and then lowering it back down to your side. Weight lifters perform this exercise with weights in their hands to strengthen the biceps muscles in the front of their arms. To maintain good form during this exercise, the arm should stay roughly at the midpoint of the trunk while curling the hand up and down. This helps the head of the arm bone, nestled in the shoulder socket, remain in its proper position with limited stress to the shoulder joint tissues.

Keeping the arm in a mechanically correct position fatigues the biceps muscles more quickly and with lighter weight. However, pushing past fatigue in order to reach a predetermined number of repetitions or lift heavier weight, the elbow compensates by rocking forward and back. When the elbow moves back, the head of the arm bone at the shoulder joint moves forward, often pulling the shoulder blade with it or stressing the tissues in the front of the shoulder. Over time this can create a host of mechanical problems in the shoulder joint.

Biceps fatigue during curls is good pain because it indicates that the muscle is being stimulated to strengthen and grow. This is what we are shooting for when performing the strengthening exercises at the end of this book. We want muscle stimulation and therefore improved strength and control of the bone or joint in question. In the biceps curl example, ignoring this fatigue to squeeze out a few more reps or allow you to lift more weight can cause shoulder joint problems. Become comfortable with and even rejoice in the fact that the muscle you are targeting is fatiguing. It is better to strengthen the muscle group incrementally rather than compensate your form—and your healing process—to squeeze out a few more repetitions. This is where bad pain comes in.

Avoidance of good pain—ignoring your body's signals—often leads to "bad" pain. Bad pain is more difficult to describe because everyone experiences it differently. It can be sharp or dull, nagging or acute. It is the pain you are trying to eliminate, the pain of injury or dysfunction. It is something you feel that you instinctively know shouldn't be happening.

You should only feel fatigue in the muscles you are targeting. Using the biceps curl example, if you feel pain at the shoulder or elbow joints while performing the curl, then you know you're experiencing bad pain. The biceps muscles are located between the shoulder and elbow joints. If you feel pain above or below the biceps muscles, it is likely that you are lifting too heavy a load or allowing your elbows to move too much. The habits that cause bad pain ultimately compromise your efforts, leading to tissue vulnerability and weakness—and more pain.

So often, clients are disappointed to find that they fatigue quickly when exercising with correct form. I happily point out that this is great news because they are finally activating and strengthening the right muscles without exacerbating their condition! Keep this in mind as you strengthen through your injury.

2 UNDERSTANDING YOUR ANATOMY

KNOWLEDGE *of any kind gets metabolized*
spontaneously and brings about a CHANGE
in AWARENESS *from where it is possible*
to create NEW REALITIES.

—DEEPAK CHOPRA

Shoulder pain can be one of the most difficult problems to fix in the body. Unless a tear or bone spur shows up on an MRI or X-ray, many health care practitioners become stumped with regards to resolving chronic or nagging shoulder and elbow pain. As you will learn, one reason for this is the shoulder's unique anatomy and mechanics, which are unlike any other joint in the body.

Shoulder and elbow problems usually come in the form of **rotator cuff** tendonitis, **bursitis**, **impingement** problems, **tennis elbow**, or **golfer's elbow**—you name it. I refer to these as **structural diagnoses** because they describe a specific painful tissue that has been injured. Typically, these diagnoses are followed up with advice to stretch, rest, or ice the involved tissue. While this may calm the irritation, an identical problem will resurface down the road or take the guise of an injury in an adjacent area. While these diagnoses pinpoint the tissues that are most affected, they don't indicate the conditions that lead to the problems in the first place. I liken this to seeing an X-ray of a broken left thumb and appropriately casting it to heal without realizing that the right hand is continually hitting it with a hammer. Until we can make the right hand stop, the left thumb will continue to be reinjured, if it ever really heals at all. Yes, the broken bone is painful, but the right hand continues to deliver more pain and injury, preventing true healing from occurring. I believe something similar is happening that causes these recurring structural issues in the body.

> **A word that ends in –itis simply means "inflammation."** For example, bursitis describes an inflamed bursa sac, epicondylitis describes an inflamed epicondyle bone of the elbow, and arthritis describes inflammation of a joint.

I interpret the presence of these structural diagnoses as evidence of **functional problems**. Functional problems are those in which muscles or joints don't move optimally and thereby create stress to the surrounding tissues. In my experience, functional problems lead to structural diagnoses and pain. This may occur due to poor movement patterns, weakness, limited range of motion, old injuries, or all of these factors. I believe the repeated stress from functional problems leads to physical changes in the body mentioned earlier such as bursitis, **arthritis**, rotator cuff tendonitis, or **epicondylitis**—in other words, structural diagnoses. Structural diagnoses, once again, don't describe the roots of the pain but instead symptoms the root problems create.

But here's the interesting thing: Pain can be eliminated even though the structural diagnosis remains. A person with shoulder bursitis can feel immediate relief when shoulder blade (scapula) function is restored. Although I don't have an MRI machine at my disposal to test this theory, I'm sure the bursitis didn't instantly resolve in this case. Instead, the irritant that caused the bursitis was corrected, allowing it to heal eventually.

Our bodies are designed to be pain free. You will see it takes very little to get yours back to working properly. The piece of the puzzle you've been missing is a more complete understanding of how things work and what you need to do to fix them. After you read this information, you will be able visualize the correct way to move as well as address the anatomical and biomechanical sources of your pain. Pain will then melt away and stay away permanently. Don't worry though, this isn't brain surgery! It's really quite simple once you've been introduced to a few key concepts.

While there are many parts to the equation, after reviewing the mechanics more closely, you will realize the simplicity of the underlying order and precision in shoulder blade and arm function. Learning about the fundamentals of shoulder and elbow movement will help you visualize exactly how they should be working throughout the day. When we are finished, you will have a complete understanding of the whys and hows behind your pain and how to fix it. To really

If you are interested in learning more about specific diagnoses, go to the **WebMD** website (www.webmd.com) or the **Family Doctor** website (www.familydoctor.org). Both are good sources of medical information.

make a difference in your life, however, you must apply this information at your workplace, sports, home, and any other environment you are in. Changing your habits will reinforce proper movement patterns which then will correct anatomical and biomechanical problems. Remember, a large part of healing yourself is visualizing ideal movement as well as knowing where you are going wrong. Your current habits, weaknesses, or deficits in range of motion are causing your pain. It will require giving your attention to your body to fix these problems. If you have little or no interest in understanding the whys and hows behind your pain, you can skip to Section 3: Corrective Exercises to get started on your program, but I don't recommend this. While these exercises will reduce or eliminate your pain, altering your habits will keep you pain free.

It's important to understand that shoulder rehabilitation and care includes a spectrum of exercise progressions. This book is designed to help you fix the underlying roots of your pain. It is not intended to offer a complete rehabilitation protocol for return to sports or exercise. However, returning to a progressive strengthening program will be more effective if you keep in mind the concepts you will learn in this book.

THE ROOTS OF SHOULDER PAIN

In the following pages you will read stories of people who suffered with shoulder or elbow pain that vanished once their shoulder blades and a few key muscles were corrected. Correcting scapular problems will be the foundation of your approach to fixing your shoulder and elbow pain.

If you have back pain or believe this may be a component of your shoulder pain, read **Fixing You: Back Pain.**

Poor back function can also lead to shoulder pain, due to the shoulder compensating for poor spinal range of motion such as with a rotated spine. For instance, I once worked with a swimmer to fix his back pain. I found his spine to be significantly rotated. I made the comment that, with a spine like his, I would expect it would be just a matter of time before his shoulder began hurting. He looked up at me and said, "My shoulder is hurting, my back just hurts more!"

If the spine is stuck in rotation to one direction, playing sports like golf, tennis, or swimming may demand more range of motion and strength from the shoulder blade. If the shoulder cannot meet these demands, pain can result. We'll assume you don't have a rotated spine or other back problem from here on.

The big picture is that anatomical changes such as tight or weak muscles create biomechanical problems such as joints not moving well; biomechanical problems cause poor movement habits, such as poor form while raising the arms overhead. These movement habits reinforce the original anatomical changes (Figure 2.1). This is a very important idea for you to keep in mind when reading this book. I will stay within this framework so you have both a big picture idea of what's happening while also understanding the details that affect it.

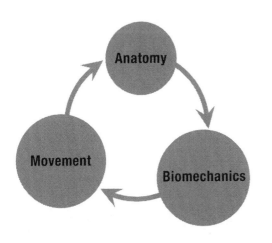

Chronic Pain Cycle
Figure 2.1 Fixing pain involves correcting each part of the pain cycle.

There are three players we will be highlighting to guide you through fixing your pain. The first is the shoulder blade (**scapula**). The scapula's function is to support the arm when it moves. The second player is the upper arm bone (**humerus**), which is affected by how much support it receives from the scapula as well as a few key muscles. The third player is the forearm whose function is largely determined by the upper arm bone as well as a couple key muscles. As you can guess, forearm movement is therefore significantly affected by the shoulder blade. So if you have tennis or golfer's elbow, don't just skip to the forearm section because everything feeds down from the scapula. Although beyond the scope of this book, it's not hard to imagine that the scapula also plays a major role in wrist and hand function by extension.

Looking Closely at Shoulder Blade Function

The shoulder joint is unique in the human body because it is a floating system of muscles, bones, ligaments, and nerves that must function nearly perfectly to be pain free. Floating? How does something float on our bodies?

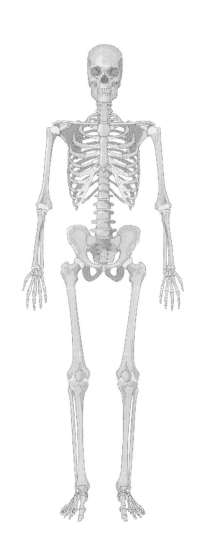

The Human Skeleton
Figure 2.2 The shoulder complex is only attached to our skeleton via the collar bone.

If you look at a human skeleton (Figure 2.2, page 36), you'll see that the bones are stacked on top of each other at almost every joint. Joint compression due to gravity is one way your body stays in alignment. But look more closely at the shoulder, and you'll see that its only connection to the rest of the skeleton is via a horizontal collarbone (**clavicle**) at the front of the rib cage. This joint acts as something of a fulcrum for shoulder function.

How can that tiny clavicle hold up the shoulder? It can't. The rest is just floating in space. What holds the shoulder in position is not joint compression but muscle tone, specifically that of the **trapezius**, **levator scapula**, **serratus anterior**, and **rhomboid** muscles as well as ligaments (Figure 2.3).

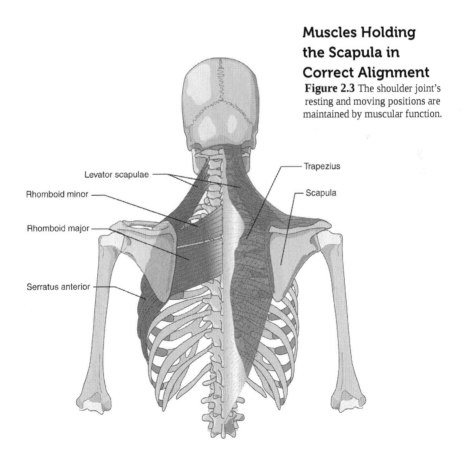

Muscles Holding the Scapula in Correct Alignment

Figure 2.3 The shoulder joint's resting and moving positions are maintained by muscular function.

Levator scapulae

Rhomboid minor

Rhomboid major

Serratus anterior

Trapezius

Scapula

This is both the beauty and curse of the shoulder joint: It has unparalleled freedom of movement, but on the other hand, it must move precisely to be pain free. Unfortunately, this is a tall order for many people. In order for the shoulder to function, the scapula must work properly, resting and moving like clockwork to keep the shoulder and elbow joints pain free.

The scapula is a strange-looking triangular bone that's slightly curved. It houses a socket into which the head of the humerus fits to form the shoulder joint (Figure 2.4). When at rest the scapula must sit at the correct height on the trunk as well as the correct distance from the spine. This sets the stage for arm movement. When the arm moves, the scapula must lift upward or elevate, rotate away from the spine, slide away from the spine (**abduct**), and finally tilt backward (**posterior tilting**). It must do this to help the arm perform whatever task it's trying to do. If the shoulder blade doesn't help the arm, then excessive stress is placed on the shoulder joint because it bears more than its share of the load. In almost every shoulder patient I see, at least a few of these functions aren't working so well.

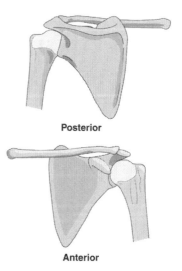

Posterior

Bones of the Shoulder Joint

Figure 2.4 The shoulder joint is formed by the upper arm bone nestling into the socket found on the scapula.

Anterior

Elevation, rotation, and abduction take place as the shoulder blade slides around on the trunk. In contrast, posterior tilting involves the scapula scooping away from the trunk. Let's talk about the sliding movements first.

One of the biggest culprits causing shoulder pain is a shoulder blade that sits too low on the trunk (depressed shoulder). When this happens, the scapula has a difficult time elevating because it must climb out of the hole it started in. It also won't rotate or abduct properly. So, for the sake of simplicity, when I speak about scapular depression, we'll assume I'm also talking about inadequate rotation, elevation, and abduction too. The figure below depicts how a normal and a depressed shoulder look at rest and overhead (Figure 2.5). The left shoulder in both pictures is in a normal position, and the right shoulder is depressed.

Ideal and Depressed Scapulae, Resting and Overhead Positions

Figure 2.5 A In the overhead position, the depressed scapula still has limited elevation, creating shoulder joint strain. **B** The left resting scapula is in a normal position while the right side is depressed.

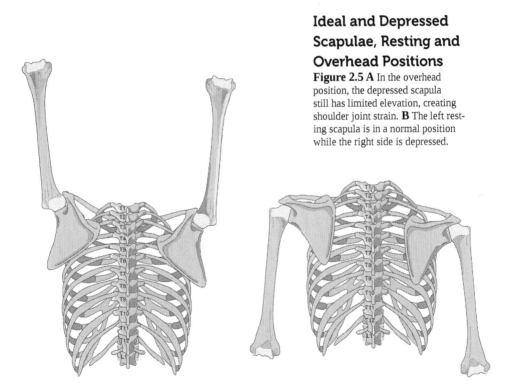

DEPRESSED SHOULDER
When the scapula sits too low on the trunk it is said to be depressed. This is usually due to lengthened or weakened upper trapezius muscles.

The client's pictures below (Figure 2.6) demonstrate what a depressed shoulder can look like in real life. Notice that her collarbones are horizontal from the front (2.6 A). Ideally, they should angle upward as your eye travels away from the center of

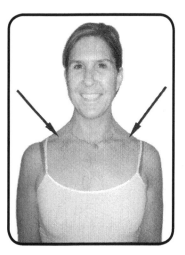

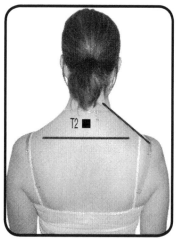

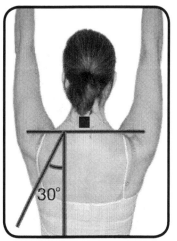

Depressed Scapula

Figure 2.6 A Front view of a woman with depressed shoulder blades. Note her collarbones are horizontal when they should be angling up toward the outside of the shoulder.

B From the back, the scapulae sit far below the desired T2 (marked) or T3 position. Also note the sharp sloping shoulder angle from the head.

C In overhead reaching the shoulder blades do not rotate, abduct or elevate adequately compromising the shoulder joint.

her chest and toward her shoulders. In the second picture (2.6 B), the shoulder blades rest far below the ideal position (marked). Do you notice the steep slope her shoulders make with her neck and head? This indicates depressed shoulders too. The inner border of the shoulder blade should also rest about three inches from the spine, which she achieves fairly well (not marked). The third picture (2.6 C) shows that the scapulae have not rotated fully with her arms in an overhead position. You can see the angle her scapulae achieves is closer to 30 degrees rather than the optimal 60 degrees of rotation that's needed to support the arms in an overhead position. Also, her shoulder blades haven't elevated up to the ideal spinal level to unload the shoulder joint.

So what's going on that depresses the shoulder blades? Well, as you can see in Figure 2.7, the trapezius and levator scapula

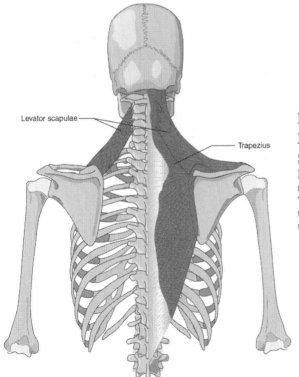

Levator scapulae

Trapezius

Muscles Elevating the Scapula

Figure 2.7 The trapezius muscle helps hold up the scapula. When it isn't performing well, the scapula may sit lower than it should on the trunk.

are designed to help hold up the shoulder blade. The trapezius should carry the bulk of the shoulder load with the levator assisting during arm raising movements. Look at how the trapezius is shaped. No other muscle in the body is quite like it!

The trapezius has three zones:

1) The upper trapezius has fibers that run up and down. It's easy to imagine these are responsible for holding the scapula in position at rest and lifting it when the arm moves.

2) The mid-trapezius has muscle fibers that run side to side. This portion controls the scapula while it rotates outward, creating a pivoting point around which it rotates.

3) The lower trapezius assists in rotating the scapula as the arm reaches upward.

Now look at the difference in size between the trapezius and the levator scapula. You'll notice the trapezius muscle is much larger and broader than the levator. Do you think the levator scapula is designed to do as much work as the trapezius? No, certainly not! But that's exactly what happens when the shoulders become depressed. Why do the shoulders become depressed in the first place? Gravity comes into play, especially with our inactive lifestyles, which allow the scapulae to gradually be pulled down. If you think about it, we rarely have opportunities to raise our arms overhead. Many ergonomic controls in industrial settings are actually designed to eliminate overhead motions—to the detriment of scapular function. As our arms work below shoulder height for longer and longer periods of time, our shoulder blades lose their fight with gravity and are pulled downward. This lengthens the trapezius, making it weaker as well.

So let's summarize: A weak or lengthened trapezius is an anatomical problem that impairs scapular movement, which is a biomechanical problem; impaired scapular movement compromises arm-raising activities and places strain on the shoulder joint, creating a movement dysfunction. Do you see how neatly that fits into our chronic pain cycle?

For women, two issues in particular contribute to depressed shoulders. The first is an ill-fitting bra with straps that are located over the outer shoulder or where the collarbone meets the scapula. This creates a long lever arm that pulls the shoulder down. To understand how this affects scapular positioning, hold your arm out to your side at shoulder height with a five-pound weight in your hand. With your arm still stretched out to the side, now put the five-pound weight on your shoulder. You'll notice it's much easier to hold the weight up when it's on your shoulder than when it's in your outstretched hand. When you're holding something up (the weight in this case), the further it is from the body, the more work it will be to maintain. The closer it is to your center, the easier it will be to hold up. Bra straps that loop over the outer shoulder rather than closer to the neck have the same effect on the scapula: They drag it down over time. This is especially important for women with large breasts. I've seen bra straps that severely dig into the shoulder from the weight they carry, pulling the shoulder blades downward. Wide straps that pass closer to the neck or cross in the back can unburden the shoulder by shortening the lever arm pulling down on the scapula, alleviating shoulder pain. Some department stores have personnel who specialize in fitting bras. When working with someone, be sure to mention your shoulder issues and the need to unload the shoulder blade as much as possible. Bringing in this book may help illustrate your needs.

The second problem particular to women is carrying a heavy bag or purse over one shoulder that drags the shoulder down, contributing to a depressed or abducted scapula. Some solutions for this include periodically switching the bag between shoulders, using bags that have double straps to disperse the weight (as in a backpack)—or simply cleaning out your bag to reduce the load.

Depressed shoulder blades can be easily corrected using the **All-Fours Rocking Stretch** (page 82) and **Wall Slides** (page 84) to stretch and strengthen the muscles responsible for getting the scapula moving.

Looking Closely at the Rotator Cuff Muscles

You can hardly talk about shoulder pain without hearing about the rotator cuff. Ever wonder why rotator cuff problems are so common? Ever wonder what the rotator cuff is? The rotator cuff muscles run from the shoulder blade to the arm bone (Figure 2.8). So what's all the hype? Why do we hear so much about the rotator cuff? Some of the rotator cuff muscles help rotate the arm bone outward (**external rotation**). They must counterbalance the muscles that turn the arm bone inward (**internal rotation**). These include other rotator cuff muscles as well as the chest and latissimus muscles that come from the trunk (Figure 2.9). The problem

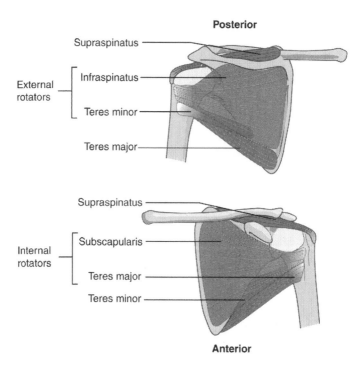

Rotator Cuff Muscles

Figure 2.8 The rotator cuff muscles attach from the scapula to the arm bone and control different movements of the arm.

is that, as you can see, the muscles turning the humerus inward are much bigger than those turning the arm bone outward, and they are also more prone to tightness. This is because most of our activities involve internally rotating our arms to work in front of us. For instance, as you're reading this book, your arms are slightly internally rotated in order to hold the book at your midline. The same goes for working on a computer or just about any task. The rotator cuff muscles' other job is to guide the head of the humerus in the shoulder socket so it doesn't slide forward too much and so that it pivots well. Think about this for a second. These muscles must do all of these things while the scapula is elevating, ro-

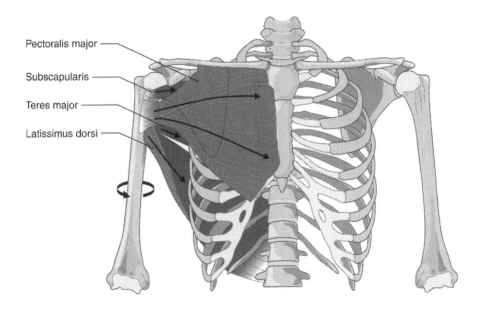

Internal Rotators of the Humerus

Figure 2.9 The muscles controlling internal rotation of the arm bone are more plentiful and larger than those controlling external rotation.

tating, abducting, and posteriorly tilting. Now you can get an idea of why the shoulder has so many problems and why it's difficult to fix these problems—well, until now, of course!

Now let's throw in a couple of 800-pound gorillas—the chest and back muscles. The **pectoralis major**, one of the chest muscles, runs from the trunk to the arm bone and contributes to internal rotation of the arm and shoulder depression when the arm raises overhead. The **latissimus dorsi**, a back muscle that begins on the pelvis and lower and mid-back, connects to the bottom corner of the scapula before it inserts onto the front of the arm bone. The latissimus also contributes to inward rotation of the arm bone. Additionally, it pulls the arm back and depresses the scapula.

If the pectoralis and latissimus are tight or overly developed, they can alter how the arm bone and/or scapula rests and moves. Again, they tend to dominate arm movements because of how we typically work with our arms and the muscles' shear size. This makes it difficult for the rotator cuff muscles to guide the head of the humerus in the shoulder socket. When this happens, the rotator cuff internal rotators also become tight, reinforcing this problem. This is often the case in weight lifters whose training emphasizes bigger or stronger chest and back muscles while excluding scapular and rotator-cuff muscles.

If you watch people who weight train frequently, you'll notice the palms of their hands face backward instead of facing into their hips when they are standing (Figure 2.10). This is caused by tight arm bone internal rotators (pectorals, latissimus, and rotator-cuff internal rotators), or a scapula that sits too far from the spine, or a combination of both. You can also see this by watching your arm as it reaches overhead. If your elbow turns out (the crease of your elbow faces in) early in the act of reaching, or if your back arches when you reach overhead, then tight internal rotators may be altering your arm movements.

When the internal rotators are dominant, the external rotators become strained from working against these enormous muscles.

Anyone who has had a massage therapist work on these rotator cuff muscles can attest to how strained and painful they can be. Stretching the internal rotators to unload stress to the external rotator muscles will be an important part of your corrective program.

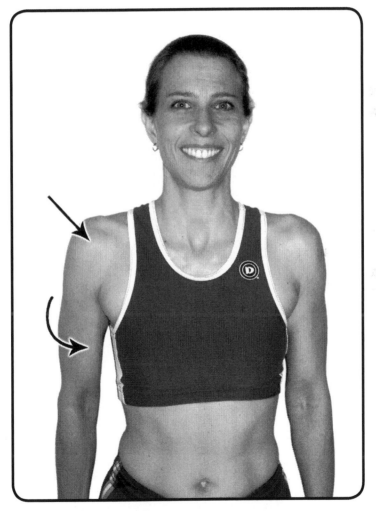

Internally Rotated Humerus

Figure 2.10 This woman's upper arm bone is excessively rotated inward. Note the crease of her right elbow faces inward while the crease of her left elbow faces forward.

ANTERIORLY GLIDED HUMERUS
Anterior glide occurs when more than 1/3 of the head of the arm bone (humerus) sits forward in the shoulder socket. This **alters the axis of rotation** and leads to injury

Finally, overdevelopment of the internal rotator muscles also contributes to the arm bone sitting too far forward (**anterior glide**) in the shoulder socket (Figure 2.11), which alters the arm bone's path of motion. The combination of an internally rotated humerus and anterior glide creates an environment where the shoulder joint throws up its hands in frustration, so to speak, because it is overwhelmed by all the forces working against it! Take a close look at those rotator cuff muscles. Notice how small they are compared to the bigger internal rotators. Those tiny rotator cuff muscles must guide the arm bone, try to hold it back in the socket, and hold their own against the overpowering goril-

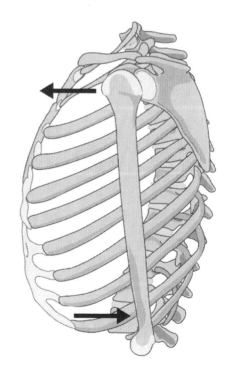

ANTERIOR GLIDE OF HUMERAL HEAD

Figure 2.11 A humeral head that sits forward in the shoulder socket is anteriorlyglided. This can result from muscle imbalances and contribute to recurring shoulder impingement issues and rotator cuff tears.

las—all while the scapula is moving beneath them! This is why it's important to periodically do activities that use your shoulders' full range of motion. That helps the muscles and joints recapture lost movement capabilities and maintain balanced muscle activation. The photographs in Figure 2.12 depict this nicely. This client's left arm worked well. She had right shoulder pain, however. This was partly due to her arm bone sitting too far forward in its socket. She learned to alter her lifting habits when exercising to work in a range of motion that wouldn't pull her arm forward. Her pain was eliminated after she gained this control. Then we gradually increased the range of motion she could work through, as well as the resistance.

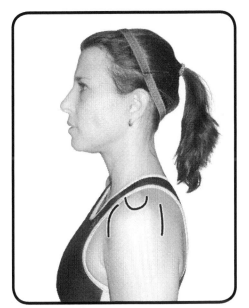 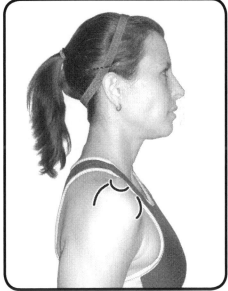

Anterior Glide of the Arm Bone

Figure 2.12 A This woman's left shoulder sits nicely in the shoulder socket. The U shape marks the acromion of the scapula. Less than 1/3 of the humeral head (outlined on the left and right) sits forward of the acromion.
B The woman's right humeral head rests too far forward out of the shoulder socket. She experiences right shoulder pain when performing upper-body exercises.

The Rotator Cuff Muscle Everyone's Talking About

One muscle is more problematic than others when it comes to shoulder pain: the **supraspinatus muscle**. When you hear people talking about rotator cuff tears or surgery, they're usually referring to the supraspinatus muscle. Tap the top of your shoulder; the bone you feel is the **acromion**, which forms the "ceiling" of the shoulder joint. As you can see in Figure 2.13, beneath the acromion is the head of the arm bone, which makes up the "floor" of the shoulder joint. The space between the floor and the ceiling is called the **subacromial space**. This is where the supraspinatus lives and works (Figure 2.14). This muscle is important for guiding the head of the humerus when you raise your arm, even if it's just a little movement.

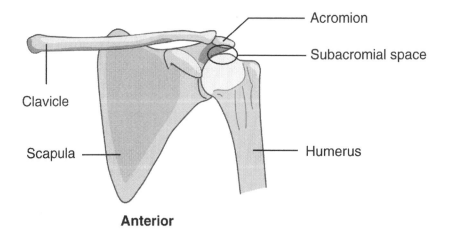

Acromion

Subacromial space

Clavicle

Scapula

Humerus

Anterior

The Subacromial Space

Figure 2.13 Note the subacromial space between the acromion and the head of the humerus. This space is necessary for the supraspinatus muscle to pass through for optimal shoulder mechanics. The supraspinatus muscle, important to shoulder function, sits in the subacromial space formed by the arm bone and the acromion. This muscle is often damaged when the subacromial space has narrowed due to poor shoulder blade mechanics.

None of us lives in a home where we bump our head on the ceiling every time we stand up. We need more space than that. The supraspinatus muscle is no different. Adequate subacromial space is necessary to allow the supraspinatus muscle to move around unencumbered. If that gap narrows, chances are the supraspinatus will come in contact with the acromion; this is referred to as impingement, which is a fancy word for pinching. Repeated impingement of this muscle can cause it to fray or eventually tear.

When your arms are down at your sides, your shoulder blade's resting position naturally maintains this gap. Remember that other scapular motion I mentioned earlier, posterior tilting? Ideally, when your arms raise overhead, your shoulder blade should tilt backward (**posterior tilt**) in addition to the sliding movements

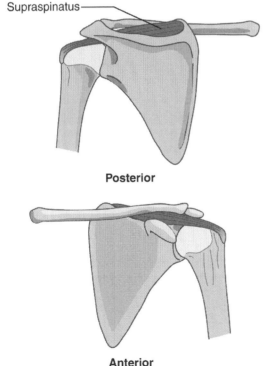

Posterior

Anterior

Back and Front Views of the Shoulder Blade with the Supraspinatus Muscle

Figure 2.14 The supraspinatus muscle, important to shoulder function, sits in the subacromial space formed by the arm bone and the acromion. This muscle is often damaged when the subacromial space has narrowed due to poor shoulder blade mechanics.

mentioned above. When the shoulder blade has sufficient posterior tilt and correctly performs its sliding movements, the subacromial space opens up and gives the supraspinatus plenty of head
room to do its thing.

Your shoulder blade tilts more effectively when you have good
posture (Figure 2.15). When you have poor or slouching posture,
the scapula can't get out of the way, which causes the supraspinatus to become pinched against the acromion (Figure 2.16). Often,
the shoulder blade doesn't tilt backward enough because it is excessively tilted forward (**anterior tilt**). Poor posture contributes to this.

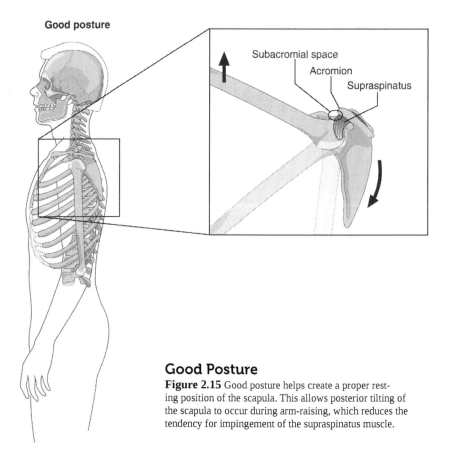

Good Posture

Figure 2.15 Good posture helps create a proper resting position of the scapula. This allows posterior tilting of
the scapula to occur during arm-raising, which reduces the
tendency for impingement of the supraspinatus muscle.

So how do we fix this? First of all, sit up straight and correct your posture! An erect posture allows your shoulder blades to tilt backward, which in turn allows your arm bones to rise higher without pinching that rotator cuff muscle. Test this yourself. Slouch in your chair and raise your arms while maintaining the slouched posture. Note how high your arms raise and if you feel any discomfort. Now sit up tall, lift your ribcage, and shrug your shoulders up while you raise your arms again. Notice that your arms can raise higher or are less restricted. Most people will find it much easier to raise their arms while maintaining the taller posture and will also find they

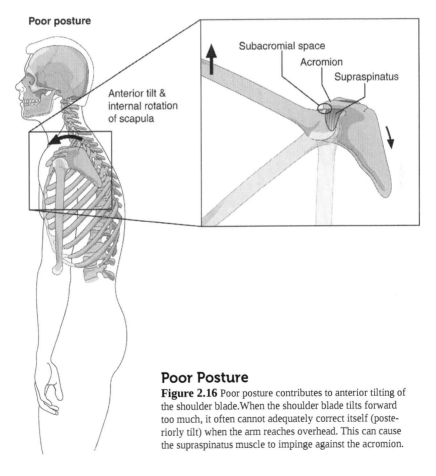

Poor Posture

Figure 2.16 Poor posture contributes to anterior tilting of the shoulder blade. When the shoulder blade tilts forward too much, it often cannot adequately correct itself (posteriorly tilt) when the arm reaches overhead. This can cause the supraspinatus muscle to impinge against the acromion.

have greater range of motion or less discomfort. When poor posture causes the humerus to prematurely bump into the acromion of the scapula, it keeps your arm from reaching its full range. Sitting up tall helps your shoulder blade tilt back and rotate out of the way. Working, resting, or playing with better posture prepares the shoulder for overhead activities and lessens microtrauma to the supraspinatus. This has enormous implications for people whose work or athletics involves reaching overhead.

You can do a lot throughout the day to correct depressed shoulders. For instance, when raising your arm overhead, visualize your scapula pushing it up, helping the arm. You can also raise the arms of your chair a little higher than normal to lift your scapula. Prop your arms up on pillows while you're working to help unload and shorten your trapezius muscle. At home, rest your arms on pillows while watching TV. Fix your posture by lifting your ribcage, creating a taller spine. This will help your scapula's posterior tilting. I've found the best way to do all this is to set up a system of reminders such as stickers on your computer, phone, clock, the dashboard of your car—anything you look at frequently. Wear a special bracelet or ring or wear your watch on the opposite wrist to remind you to periodically check in on your shoulder position.

I once saw a patient for rehab after a rotator cuff surgical repair. She had a sedentary job and didn't participate in sports or exercise regularly. When I asked how she tore her muscle, she related that it happened when she was lifting her suitcase into the overhead bin on an airplane as she was leaving for a much-needed vacation. How tragic! I believe her poor posture at work was reinforced by a slumped posture while watching TV at home. Other than getting some food out of her cupboards, she rarely raised her arms overhead. She never gave her shoulder blades a chance to move out of their anterior-

> Performing even a single repetition of **Wall Slides** (page 84) will help **restore proper range of motion** to your shoulders.

ly tilted or depressed posture; they just couldn't comply when she needed them to. We all need our arms to reach overhead at one time or another. Doesn't it make sense to prepare for that, even a little bit, by sitting up taller?

Performing the **Hand On Head** exercise (page 105) at various times during the day is very effective for **retraining the scapula to elevate properly**.

We covered a lot of information here! Let's take a breather, step back, and recap. Internal rotator muscles in the arm bone can become tight (an anatomical change); this muscle tightness alters how the arm bone rotates and rests in the shoulder socket (a biomechanical change), which can make the arm bump into the roof of the shoulder too soon during arm raising (a movement dysfunction). Add a depressed scapula to the mix together with poor posture, and we have a formula for shoulder pain.

Let's put it all together: A depressed shoulder blade doesn't adequately support a moving arm bone that is internally rotated too much (which may be due in part to tight internal rotator muscles). Poor posture prevents the shoulder blade from tilting or sliding out of the way, which causes the arm bone to prematurely bump the supraspinatus muscle against the roof of the shoulder. All the while, the poor little rotator cuff muscles are trying to control this mess but are overworked and strained from the effort! And you were wondering why you had shoulder pain! Of course there are variances in this model. Sometimes the scapular depression plays a bigger role than the internal rotator tightness or postural problems. But usually there is some component of all three of these issues.

Client Connection: Barbara's Bum Shoulder

Barbara was a fit thirtysomething, an avid rock climber and computer programmer who had surgery on her right shoulder two years prior to fix her shoulder pain. The surgery was somewhat successful, but she still had pain in the front of her shoulder. She was unable to climb or strength train because of it. She had been to several people for help but to no avail.

I assessed her shoulder (using the landmarks discussed in "Landmarks and Solutions for Proper Shoulder Function," page 57) and found that her right scapula was sitting too close to her spine. It sat approximately two inches from the spine rather than the ideal three inches. Looking at her other shoulder landmarks, we discovered that her scapula did not rotate enough or slide out from her spine when her arm was overhead. These movements are critical for anyone—and definitely for a rock climber.

The Fixing You Approach for Impaired Shoulder Blade Function

I love to mention Barbara because her solution was so simple it surprised us both. I simply asked her to allow her scapula to rest another inch away from her spine. Once I showed her where the three-inch mark was, I asked her to raise her arms overhead.

"No pain," she said surprised. "Wow! You mean it was that simple?"

We took Barbara through an arm weight-training routine. Every time she experienced shoulder pain, we found she had allowed her scapula to squeeze back toward her spine again. Each time I showed her where it should be, her pain disappeared.

"But it feels like my arm is too far from my body," she offered.

"What's 'normal' by your standards isn't correct. You must relearn your sense of where your shoulder should be," I replied. This highlights an important point. If your brain thinks your body should move one way, but your body is telling you something else, listen to your body.

The only other exercise I gave her was the All-Fours Rocking Stretch exercise because her strength and range of motion were both good. The All-Fours Rocking Stretch exercise helped her shoulder blade move through the range of motion it needed to remain pain free.

"I can't believe after all these years and the doctors and therapists I've seen, it could be this simple!" she said when she returned a week later.

I smiled because it confirmed to me that as long as we follow the few simple rules of how the shoulder blade needs to move, pain usually melts away. Barbara was already climbing again. Every time she felt pain, she allowed that shoulder to relax outward and her pain would disappear.

Hopefully you noticed that treating Barbara's shoulder-joint pain had nothing to do with directly addressing the shoulder joint and everything to do with restoring shoulder blade mechanics. Once the scapula moves and stabilizes well, stress to the shoulder joint diminishes and tissue healing can occur.

LANDMARKS AND SOLUTIONS FOR PROPER SHOULDER FUNCTION

So where are your shoulder blades supposed to rest? There are precise rules, or landmarks, for this. These landmarks help determine how the shoulder and elbow function. Restoring shoulder function to reach these ideal positions eliminates most shoulder and elbow pain. Your scapula needs to move properly to unload the shoulder joint. It's supposed to elevate, rotate, and abduct to keep all the players happy. Just about every shoulder or elbow client I see has problems with these basic movements.

In my experience, there is rarely just one landmark that's deficient. Especially if a resting position landmark is off, the stage is set for dysfunction when the arm moves. Restoring correct movement patterns can be a very quick process. I've had clients with only 30 degrees of scapular rotation reach 55 degrees in one session and eliminate their pain. The exercises outlined in this book are designed to correct these landmarks and therefore shoulder and elbow function.

Assessing your shoulder landmarks can be tricky but important for understanding the big picture of shoulder function.

I recommend you find a physical therapist to help you with this. All of these assessments can be viewed at our website at **www.FixingYou.net**. Type in the code at the back of this book to access the video clips.

Landmark 1: Scapula resting at T2 or T3

The top of the shoulder blade should sit roughly at the second (T2) or third (T3) **thoracic vertebra** (Figure 2.17). I often see scapulae that sit lower than this. When this occurs, the upper tra-

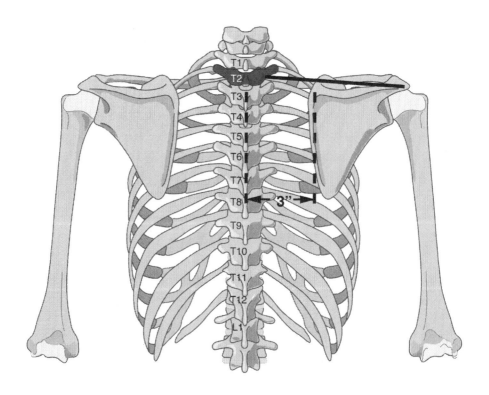

Landmarks for Resting Shoulder Position

Figure 2.17 A shoulder at rest should have its vertebral border approximately 3 inches from the spine. The top of the scapula should align with T2 or T3.

pezius is typically too long and/or weak to hold up the scapula. I see this problem in nearly everyone with shoulder or elbow pain. Shoulder blades sitting too low (depressed) set the stage for inadequate elevation of the scapula during overhead motions, compromising shoulder muscles and other tissues.

Exercise Recommendations: The All-Fours Rocking Stretch, Wall Slides, and Hand on Head are useful exercises to help correct this. Other exercises could include Latissimus Dorsi Stretch and Side-Lying Arm Slides.

Daily Tip: Try this simple movement to train your upper trapezius to work better: Shrug your shoulder up as your arm reaches overhead, and allow it to remain up while the arm lowers (this also helps with neck pain; see *Fixing You: Neck Pain & Headaches*). This elevates the shoulder blade until the upper trapezius muscle is adequately retrained. If you have a depressed scapula, prop up your elbows on pads to elevate your shoulders while driving, working, or resting at home.

Landmark 2: Scapula border 3 inches from the spine

The vertical border of the scapula closest to the spine (**vertebral border**) needs to be approximately three inches from the spine (Figure 2.17). This is true whether you're five feet tall or seven feet tall. I see problems in both directions, either too close to the spine or too far away, but usually one or both scapulae sit too far away from the spine.

Exercise Recommendations: The Trapezius Strengthening exercise is helpful to correct an abducted scapula. Also, when performing Wall Slides or the All-Fours Rocking Stretch, begin by squeezing your shoulder blades together to achieve the biomechanically correct position three inches from the spine.

Daily Tip: During the day, monitor whether your shoulders are becoming too rounded and squeeze them gently together (or relax them outward if they are sitting too close to the spine) until you achieve the three-inch position from the spine. It will take a little time to learn how to find this corrected position, but you will master it quickly. When driving, move your seat one notch closer to the steering wheel. Keeping your shoulder blades in contact with the seat can help them avoid excessive abduction.

Landmark 3: Scapular rotation at 60 degrees

The shoulder blade needs to rotate outward about 60 degrees when the arm is in an overhead position (Figure 2.18). I often see scapulae with only 30 to 40 degrees of rotation. Inadequate rotation means the arm is not supported properly when moving into overhead positions and can lead to shoulder strain. When the scapula stops rotating, the arm bone must continue the movement against the fixed scapula, creating excessive motion at the shoulder joint. Excessive motion at any joint typically causes pain.

Exercise Recommendations: To help correct poor scapular rotation, do the All-Fours Rocking Stretch. Wall Slides, Trapezius Strengthening, Arm Waves, Side-Lying Arm Waves, and the Latissimus Dorsi Stretch are also useful.

Daily Tip: When raising your arm, visualize reaching up with your shoulder blade instead of with your hand. You will get the same result—your hand being overhead—but it will feel completely different. This is because you are using the scapular muscles to help lift your arm rather than letting your shoulder muscles do all the work. This will help mobilize the scapula, activating key muscles that have been lying dormant. Again, this movement will initially feel awkward or unnatural to you. This is because your movement habits have created a perception of "natural movement" that's inaccurate and needs to be retrained.

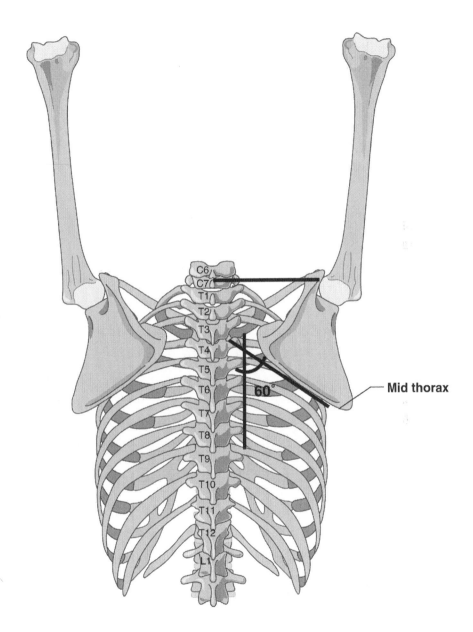

Landmarks for Overhead Shoulder Position

Figure 2.18 In the overhead position, ideally the scapula should rotate 60 degrees, elevate to approximately C7, and abduct to the mid-trunk.

Landmark 4: Inferior angle of the scapula at mid-trunk

The bottom corner of the scapula, the **inferior angle**, needs to reach approximately the midpoint of the rib cage on the side of the trunk (Figure 2.18, page 61). I frequently see the inferior angle fall short of this mark reaching only the back of the rib cage. This usually happens because of poor scapular rotation.

Exercise Recommendations: To help correct this, do the All-Fours Rocking Stretch and Wall Slides.

Daily Tip: Again, visualize reaching up with your shoulder blade instead of your hand when reaching overhead. Your shoulder blade will slide away from your spine in response to this. Put your finger on the midpoint of the side of your trunk as a target, and reach overhead while trying to touch your finger with your scapula.

Landmark 5. Scapula elevation to C7

The upper, outer edge of the scapula needs to elevate to approximately to C7, the seventh **cervical vertebra** (Figure 2.18, page 61). Especially when the scapula is depressed to begin with, the chances of reaching C7 are much reduced. When the scapula does not elevate properly, increased stress is placed on the shoulder muscles, which leads to impingement or tears. This is often at the root of shoulder and elbow pain.

Exercise Recommendations: The All-Fours Rocking Stretch, Wall Slides, and Hand On Head exercises are useful to help correct this.

Daily Tip: To train your upper trapezius to work better, elevate your shoulder as your arm reaches overhead; visualize reaching up with your scapula instead of with your hand. Allow your scapula to remain raised while your arm lowers. When sitting, prop your elbows up so your shoulders elevate.

Client Connection: Gary's Gliding Arm

Gary had shoulder pain for 20 years, since playing college football and baseball. It would die down when he stopped lifting weights and then re-emerge when he tried to exercise again. He was a muscular athlete who wanted to continue weight training and playing sports but couldn't get past his chronic shoulder pain. After evaluating his shoulder, I found his shoulder blade sat too low on his trunk (depressed) and too far away from his spine (abducted), and his arm bone (humerus) was rotated in too much (internal rotation) as well as sitting too far forward in the shoulder socket (anterior glide). Furthermore, his shoulder was limited in almost all ranges of motion. Gary had three issues to contend with: a shoulder blade that sat too low and too far away from the spine, an arm bone that was rotated inward, and an arm bone that sat too far forward out of the shoulder socket.

The central issue was that his shoulder blade was not resting where it should and therefore wasn't moving correctly either. This affects all other arm functions. That's because the shoulder blade's purpose is to support the arm during movement. If the scapula moves incorrectly, then the shoulder joint must carry a larger burden. It can do this for only so long before tissues become worn out or painful.

The other issue was the muscles Gary worked so hard to develop, actually became part of the problem. Remember Figure 2.9 (page 45) and all those muscles rotating the arm bone inward? When they are overly tight, they set up the shoulder joint for biomechanical problems and pain. When they are overly tight or dominant, they rotate the arm bone inward, setting the shoulder joint up for movement problems and pain. These same muscles limit arm bone and even shoulder blade range of motion.

I've found that correcting range of motion is usually the best place to start. You want the shoulder to be able to move the way it's supposed to before adding strengthening exercises. In Gary's case, we targeted both his arm and scapula using Wall Slides and the All-Fours Rocking Stretch because these gentle yet powerful exercises restore range of motion.

The All-Fours Rocking Stretch serves the dual purposes of stretching key muscles in the arm and scapula as well as guiding these bones to restore proper movement patterns. This single exercise is a real workhorse for fixing shoulder pain and will most likely be one you will perform in a maintenance program. When performing the All-Fours Rocking Stretch exercise, pay special attention to whether your elbow crease rotates in while rocking back onto your heels (this is demonstrated in the video clip online at **www.FixingYou.net**). This indicates tightness of your internal rotator muscles. Stretching them simply means not allowing the arm bone to rotate while rocking back. This may initially be painful; if so, stop at the point of pain or allow the elbow crease to rotate in just enough to ease the pain. As these muscles stretch, you will be able to rock back further onto your heels before pain begins. Eventually there will be no pain.

We also began with Wall Slides. This exercise uses gravity for resistance and is therefore considered a strengthening exercise to some degree. This exercise is important to teach the shoulder blade and arm to move together in proper sequence during overhead motions.

While exercising, sink the head of the arm bone back into the socket and feel it stay there during exercise. For instance, biceps curls is a common exercise that contributes to the arm bone sliding forward in the shoulder socket. Reduce the weight until you are able to maintain the curl without allowing your shoulder to slide forward.

After Gary could perform these exercises without pain, we added the Trapezius Strengthening exercise. This exercise targets key muscles that help move and stabilize the scapula as the arm moves. Most people with shoulder pain have weak scapular rotators and stabilizers, which this strengthening exercise helps correct.

Finally, we layered on the last exercise to correct his arm bone, which sat too far forward in his shoulder socket. Prone Arm Waves is an excellent exercise to help draw the head of the arm bone back into the socket or at least add some stability to front of the shoulder. The most powerful method to correct his anteriorly glided arm bone was to ask him not to allow it to slide forward while exercising. With a little bit of focus, he was able to master this quickly.

Permanently fixing Gary's shoulder pain involved making him aware of his movement impairments that contributed to his anatomical and biomechanical problems. I asked Gary to resist the temptation to allow his arm to rotate in and to involve his scapulae more during arm-raising activities. These two simple instructions reinforced all his exercises.

Looking Closely at the Forearm and Elbow

So far, we've paid a lot of attention to the shoulder blade and arm bone. You've learned that when the shoulder blade doesn't rest or move as it's designed to, there is a good chance the arm bone will also have problems. If the arm bone is rotated inward, then the forearm will have problems. These problems have to do with how well the forearm rotates into a hand-down position (**pronation**) and a hand-up position (**supination**). Both of these motions are extremely important because we use them all the time during work and play. Forearm rotation is important to wrist and hand function because we need to rotate our forearm to type, cook, dress, play sports, or pretty much anything else.

As you will see, the forearm and upper arm bone are functionally entwined. If the upper arm bone is rotated inward, then the forearm will also usually rotate inward too much. The forearm muscles responsible for this rotation then become shortened from disuse while the others responsible for the opposite rotation become lengthened from overuse. So let's get familiar with some basic anatomy of the elbow, so you can see how these parts work together.

The elbow joint is composed of three bones. Two of those bones, the **radius** and **ulna**, belong to the forearm; the humerus is the third bone. The forearm muscles attach to bony bumps on the inner and outer portions of the humerus at the elbow joint. These bumps are the **epicondyles**. The muscles that control rotation of your forearm—the pronators that rotate your forearm into the hand-down position, and the supinators that rotate your forearm into the hand-up position—attach to the epicondyles. The pronators and supinators lie deeper than other muscles that control the wrist and hand movements, which also connect at the epicondyles. You can see in Figure 2.19 that the **pronator teres** muscle originates at both the ulna bone and inner (medial) epicondyle and inserts onto the radius bone. The **pronator quadratus** is found closer to the wrist and connects the radius and ulna. The **supinator muscle** originates on the outer (lateral) epicondyle and inserts onto the radius. This muscle group helps rotate your

Deep Forearm
Rotator Muscles
Figure 2.19 The deep forearm muscles responsible for rotation of the forearm are typically tight in people with elbow pain. Tightness can contribute to elbow and hand dysfunction.

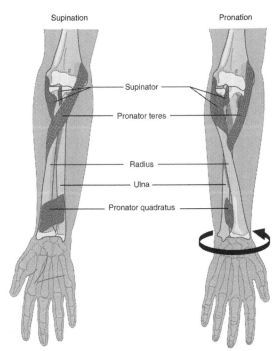

palm up. Both groups of rotator muscles must work in concert to exert fine control on forearm rotation, so your wrist and hand can function precisely. Your forearm should rotate 80 to 90 degrees in both directions (with palm up or palm down). Essentially, if your elbow is resting on a table, your wrist bones should be able to lie flat. In my experience, elbow pain begins when forearm rotation is compromised.

When the arm bone becomes rotated inward due to muscle tightness or scapular problems mentioned above, the forearm rotates downward (pronation). The forearm muscles controlling this motion—the pronators—will then shorten because their full range of motion is no longer used or needed. When the pronators get short and tight, the muscles opposing forearm pronation, the supinators, lengthen to compensate. These adaptations (anatomical changes) affect the function of muscles that bend and straighten the wrist because now the forearm is relatively rotated while these muscles are working.

The muscles that bend and straighten the wrist have their origins at the elbow. Altering their function often leads to tennis or golfer's elbow. The medical term for tennis elbow is **lateral epicondylitis**, and for golfer's elbow it's **medial epicondylitis**. Both of these terms simply mean that inflammation is present either at the outer (lateral) bone of the elbow or the inner (medial) bone of the elbow. These terms do not specify what is inflamed or why. Traditional treatment is aimed at the superficial muscles of the elbow joint that flex and extend the wrist and fingers. Although these muscles may be painful, I believe the actual problem lies in the deeper muscles that control rotation of the forearm. Look again at where the forearm rotator muscles insert (the pronator teres and supinator; see Figure 2.19), and you'll see they're perfectly positioned to cause this irritation. I have also found similar deficits in people with carpal tunnel syndrome, thoracic outlet syndrome, and generalized wrist or hand pain. Improving forearm rotation reduces stress where the muscles insert at the elbow and on the other muscles that must compensate for their lack of movement.

Client Connection: Trent's Tennis Elbow

My treatment for tennis elbow used to involve painful digging into the forearm muscles to work out knots in the muscles that cause pain. However, the pain would always return. When Trent, a 32-year-old software engineer, came in with right elbow pain, I decided I needed to find a better solution. He had undergone surgery that severed a major forearm muscle about two years prior to meeting me. This was the very muscle I typically worked on to treat tennis elbow. If it was severed, then it couldn't be the culprit!

Before the surgery, Trent could not lift his right hand to his mouth without suffering excruciating pain. When I first started working with him, he could lift his hand to his mouth without pain but could do little else. Trent was a golfer and lifted weights. He had a golf game with an important client coming up in about eight weeks. He needed to play.

We assessed Trent's shoulder and found the right shoulder blade sat too low on the trunk (depressed) as well as too far out from the spine (abducted). Are you noticing a pattern? We performed several other tests and found that his trapezius muscles, which move and stabilize the shoulder blades, were weak. He also lacked range of motion, necessary for the right arm bone to move well.

Because Trent's goal was to play golf again, I put a club in his hand and watched his swing. Then, I looked a little more carefully at his elbow function in relation to his shoulder. When I made his shoulder move through the proper range of motion, there was a change in the club head angle. I decided to test the forearm rotation; it was diminished. As discussed earlier, the forearm should rotate 80 to 90 degrees into both palm-up (supination) and palm-down (pronation) positions. Trent was missing approximately 20 degrees in the first direction (palm up) and 30 degrees in the second (palm down). This was due to tight forearm rotator muscles.

The Fixing You Approach for Tennis Elbow

We addressed Trent's shoulder function by first restoring proper range of motion to the shoulder blade and arm bone (All-Fours Rocking Stretch and Arm Waves). We then layered on advanced range-of-motion and strengthening exercises (Wall Slides and Trapezius Strengthening). Although Trent's elbow was his primary complaint, after working with his shoulder he realized that he had some major deficits to correct there as well.

To address Trent's forearm range of motion, I developed a forearm stretch into both palm-down and palm-up directions (Assisted Forearm Stretch). We did this while Trent stabilized his shoulder blade in a corrected position according to the landmarks discussed earlier. Once we improved his forearm rotation, I asked him to hold the golf club again.

"Oh my god!" he exclaimed. "There's hardly any pain!"

The goal isn't "hardly any pain"; the goal is to be pain free, so we assessed his elbow again, this time while he was holding the club. His forearm had rotated again, which forced his shoulder blade to slide out in order to get his forearm into a proper position to swing his club.

> **Restoring forearm rotation** together with scapula correction has proven to be highly effective when **fixing tennis or golfer's elbow.**

We stretched his forearm again.

"No pain," he said, stunned. "I can't believe it!"

He took some swings while we adjusted his shoulder and showed him how to monitor his forearm position. The swings were pain free. I developed exercises to maintain the forearm's range of motion in his at-home exercise program (Forearm Rotational Stretching exercise).

Our next step was to strengthen the forearm muscles while maintaining the forearm range of motion. Trent could not handle the impact of the club against the ball without pain. So I devised a stretch/strengthening exercise (Assisted Forearm Rotational

Strengthening) in which I slowly rotated the club while he gently resisted, keeping his shoulder in proper alignment. The exercise moves the forearm through its full range of motion in both directions (supination and pronation) while strengthening the muscles. We practiced this for a couple sessions, and then it was time for a test run.

He was naturally reluctant to get out and hit a bucket of balls, but I convinced him that if he didn't experience pain in the clinic, then he shouldn't out on the driving range. Also, the important business-related golf outing was getting close, and he needed to be able to play. We both needed to know whether this was really working.

Trent came back in the next week. "I did what you asked. I hope you're happy now," he started.

I was a little unsettled. "So what happened?" I asked.

He paused. "I hit 10 balls on Friday. It felt good so I hit another 10. Still no problems, so I hit another 10. Then I thought, 'Rick would want me to stop at this point to see if there is any latent soreness,' but I couldn't. So I went out and played a round," he said.

"So then what?" I asked, concerned.

"I had the best game I've had in years," he beamed. "No pain!"

That was Trent's last visit. I ran into him two years later—and he still had no elbow pain.

TESTING 1, 2, 3...

To test your forearm rotation, place your shoulder blades at about three inches from your spine and at approximately T2 or T3 (refer to "Landmarks and Solutions for Proper Shoulder Function," page 57). Next, simply place your elbows at your sides, bent at 90 degrees with your thumbs pointing up toward the ceiling, and stabilize your shoulder blades so your upper arm does not move (Figure 2.20 A, page 71). Rotate your hands so your palms are facing down (pronated) as in Figure 2.20 B. Look at your wrist bones. Are they completely rotated? Did your elbows slightly slide away from your trunk while you did this? Was it difficult to

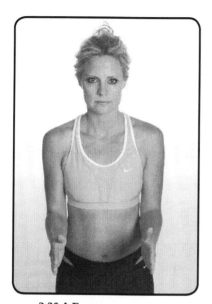

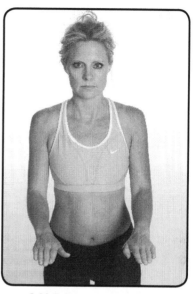

2.20 A Forearm assesment,
start position

2.20 B Forearm pronation

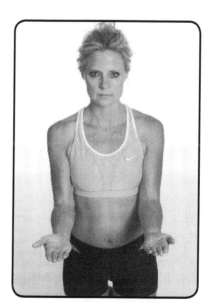

2.20 C Forearm supination

Forearm Assesment

Figure 2.20 The forearm range-of-motion test involves rotating forearm into pronation and supination while the shoulders are in correct anatomical position. Be care-
ful not to allow your elbows to move while rotating yourß forearms.

maintain the correct scapular position? If so, retest without allowing your elbows to move and with your shoulder blade stabilized.

Don't measure rotation based on whether your hand is palm down, as your hand can rotate further after the wrist has stopped. Instead, use the wrist bones as your guide. I like to use a ruler that sits across both wrist bones to help me see what's going on. If you see the ruler isn't horizontal after testing, then the rotator muscles are likely too short and forearm rotation has been compromised. Also upper arms and/or shoulders that aren't properly positioned or stabilized can give a false result.

Next, rotate your hands so your palms are facing up (supinated) as in Figure 2.20 C. Again, check your wrist's angle, not your palm's angle, using the ruler as your guide. Did your elbows slide toward your trunk while testing this motion? If so, retest with your arm bone and shoulder blade stabilized.

How did you do? Did you find that you had to work hard to control your shoulder blade and elbow while testing? If so, chances are your forearm's rotator muscles are tight and need to be stretched, even if your forearm was able to rotate fully. Try the Assisted Forearm Stretch exercise on page 87.

Client Connection: Eldon's Elbow Pain

Eldon was a 45-year-old software technician who had elbow pain for three years. It was so bad that he couldn't straighten his right elbow. He had been to a therapist who managed to straighten it out, but he still had terrible shooting pain every time he straightened or bent his elbow. After a few repetitions it would loosen up and stop hurting. He couldn't fully rotate his right forearm in either palm-up (supination) or palm-down (pronation) directions. When his palm turned down, I noticed his right shoulder slipped forward. This was not good news for someone working on computers because he worked all day long in the palm down position while typing.

I evaluated Eldon and found that his shoulder sat too low on his trunk (depressed) and too far out to the side (abducted). His range of motion was also poor in some key shoulder muscles that allow the arm to move independently of the shoulder blade.

The Fixing You Approach for Elbow Pain

We addressed Eldon's shoulder problems by focusing first on range-of-motion exercises to correct scapula movement (All-Fours Rocking Stretch) and shoulder range of motion (Arm Waves). Eldon still had pain in his elbow when he moved it. So during his next visit, we layered on the Trapezius Strengthening and Wall Slides exercises. We retested his elbow: It still hurt.

During his third visit, once I was sure his shoulder's range of motion and strength were adequate, we performed the Assisted Forearm Stretch exercise while Eldon held his shoulder in the correct position. Then we tested the elbow—and this time, no pain. Later in the session Eldon said his elbow had started to hurt again. I looked at his shoulder blade and saw that it had slid out too far again. I asked him to squeeze it back to the desired three inches from the spine, and his elbow pain disappeared. Learning to hold his scapula in the correct position was the key to permanently fix this problem.

Eldon's solution was a combination of restoring proper shoulder blade strength and position as well as forearm range of motion. Now whenever Eldon's elbow begins to hurt, he automatically slightly squeezes in his shoulder blade. Usually, the elbow pain will go away. If it doesn't, then he performs the forearm stretches found in Section 3: Corrective Exercises.

Client Connection: Georgia's Gripe About Her Grip

Georgia was a hardworking woman in her 40s who had experienced severe right elbow pain for a few months. She was right-handed and came in wearing a tennis elbow strap on her forearm. She told me it eased the pain a bit but it always returned. Georgia cleaned houses and played golf, and she couldn't grip her supplies or clubs without terrible pain.

Table 2.1

Grip	L (lbs.)	R Pain (lbs.)	R Max (lbs.)
#1	30	15	20
#2	70	45	60
#3	75	35	40
#4	52	25	30
#5	55	25	35

Table 2.1 The lower the grip position number means closer approximation of fingers to palm. Left maximum grip in pounds is shown in the second column. The third column shows the poundage where pain was felt with the right hand and then the maximum strength possible with the right hand (fourth column) with pain.

Table 2.2

Grip	L (lbs.)	R Pain (lbs.)	R Max (lbs.)
#1	33	20	20
#2	72	50	65
#3	75	45	60
#4	55	50	65
#5	57	40	45

Table 2.2. Grip testing after one minute of forearm stretching.

I assessed her shoulder and asked her to hold it in a correct position while I tested her grip strength. Table 2.1 shows her right hand strength compared to that of her left hand. I asked her to stop when the pain began on the right and then squeeze through the pain to give me her maximum grip strength.

I then stretched her right forearm into both pronation and supination for approximately one minute in each direction (Assisted Forearm Stretch). We retested her strength and pain level with her shoulder in the correct position, which is represented in Table 2.2.

Although this is hardly a stringent testing environment, the results were dramatic. I gave Georgia the Forearm Rotational Stretching exercise for homework as well as exercises to correct her shoulder blade's range of motion and positioning (All-Fours Rocking Stretch and Arm Waves). During our next appointment, Georgia told me she had no more elbow pain while working or playing golf. Although she responded very well, I gave her the Trapezius Strengthening and Wall Slides exercises to reinforce the new shoulder blade dynamics.

Let's put all of this together so you can see the big picture. The scapula has a lot to do with forearm and elbow pain because it affects the arm bone's position; the arm bone affects the forearm's position. Fixing the scapula is usually a big part of eliminating elbow pain. Once your scapular mechanics are corrected, you can focus on your forearm, which may be too tight in terms of rotation in either direction. The simple stretching exercise I devised to correct this is fast and effective (Assisted Forearm Stretch, page 87), except you'll need someone to help you. It's really quite simple when you boil it down like this!

Get a Good Night's Sleep

In almost all cases, if I can help someone sleep at night without pain, healing will occur at a much faster pace. Essentially, this boils down to experimenting with propping up or supporting your arm, shoulder, or wrist with towels or pillows to relieve stress to your shoulder or elbow. When doing so, begin with your favorite sleeping position as this is the one you are most likely to return to while asleep. Try the following recommendations to fix your sleeping habits:

Lying on your side makes your bottom shoulder slide forward underneath you (abduction). This should be avoided—especially if you've found that your scapula is sitting too far from your spine. The best way to manage this is to try to position the scapula underneath and behind you, so it doesn't slide forward. If that fails, try sleeping on the other side and resting your top arm on a pillow to prevent excessive shoulder blade abduction.

If you are used to sleeping on the painful shoulder, then experiment by propping up the affected side's wrist on pillows (bringing it off the bed) and note whether this decreases your pain. This essentially brings it into more **internal rotation** and should reduce stress to the shoulder joint.

When sleeping on your back, tight chest muscles or biceps muscles can pull your arm bone forward in your shoulder socket, contributing to an anterior glide. To reduce this stress and correct this, place your arm on a pillow.

If you sleep on your stomach, place pillows underneath each shoulder to reduce the forward pull of gravity. This will also put the head of the humerus in a better position in the shoulder socket.

3 CORRECTIVE EXERCISES

I've been a few places like that where I've thought, "A BREAKTHROUGH *is possible here. This is the place for the* EXERCISES *that will bring me to* WHERE I WANT TO BE.*"

—JOSEPH CAMPBELL

Most of the shoulder problems I see fit into similar patterns (depressed and/or abducted scapula with internally rotated humerus or an anterior glide) and are helped by regularly performing a core group of exercises. There are many combinations of other potential problems; however, it is not within the scope of this book to explain all possible movement dysfunctions. Also, this is not meant to serve as a progressive strengthening program for people with these injuries, although if you follow the principles that have eliminated your pain, you should have a firm handle on exactly what will be good and what will be harmful in your exercise progression.

Resist the temptation to push too far too fast, and remember to **listen to your body**. If you feel pain, stop!

These exercises require attention to precision to get them right. You'll find that some of the exercises are difficult or even seem impossible at first. That means you need them, so stick with them. The stretching exercises are generally held for 30 to 60 seconds. Performing two to five repetitions is usually all that's needed to experience a positive effect. During the first week, I typically ask my clients to commit to performing their stretches as often as possible (two to five times each day) to aggressively reduce their symptoms. It should always feel good to perform the stretching exercises, so this really shouldn't be a hard sell. After the first week, when your symptoms have abated,

Poor form or posture during strength training can promote shoulder pain. Understand your poor habits and **counter them with good form.**

you can ease off and find the ideal number of times needed to keep your pain at bay. I recommend doing the exercises first thing in the morning and last thing before bed as most people's pain becomes aggravated during sleep.

After the stretching phase, begin strengthening. Add one exercise at a time to focus on getting it right and to test whether your pain is made worse by a particular movement. If your pain worsens, then your technique is incorrect or it is not the right exercise for you. Pay attention to how you are performing the exercise. Read the instructions carefully, and watch the video clips on the Fixing You website at **www.FixingYou.net**. Once you are successfully performing one exercise, then add the next. Each time you add a new strengthening exercise, don't change anything else about your program. This way, if you experience pain, you can isolate which exercise may be the cause. Strengthening exercises are performed similarly, five to ten repetitions for one to two sets or until fatigue or compensatory movements occur. For instance, when doing the Wall Slides exercise, your arm may rotate inward; this is a compensatory movement. If this occurs, either stop the exercise or try to do it without allowing the arm to internally rotate.

> **If you are weight training,** you may find that you must **temporarily decrease the weight** you are using. It's okay—fixing your shoulder and/or elbow is the **bigger picture.**

This is where your attention really comes in. The strengthening exercises are meant to strengthen specific muscles and, of course, be pain free. For example, when performing Wall Slides, we are generally targeting upper trapezius strength as well as promoting scapular rotation, elevation, and abduction. So if you feel fatigue in your shoulders or biceps or feel pain in your neck, then you should stop and pay attention to your form. You should feel the effort in the upper trapezius, between your shoulder and your neck—and you should not feel pain in your shoulder after the exercise because it is designed to eliminate pain, not trigger it. So take a moment to visualize the muscles you are attempting to train.

Another method that works well for my clients is to rapidly and briskly tap the muscle we are targeting. Sticking with the Wall Slides example, you can rapidly tap the upper trapezius muscle, located between your shoulder and your neck to "wake it up." Feel whether it has become harder due to its contraction. Keep tapping it to connect your consciousness to the muscle and develop your awareness of it and get it firing.

Just a little bit of strengthening will effect a positive change. As always, quality is more important than quantity. Strengthening exercises only need to be performed two to three times a day initially, although the Hand On Head exercise can be performed throughout the day to relieve symptoms and retrain the trapezius muscle. Once your pain diminishes and your habits are corrected, you may only need to perform the strengthening exercises once a day, once a week, once a month, or perhaps never again when your corrected movement habits are strengthening your muscles as needed, feeding your body rather than breaking it down.

The exercises that give my clients the most bang for the buck are listed on the following page. All are critical to restore proper shoulder function. Begin with those focusing on shoulder and elbow range of motion; once you have mastered them, then progress to strengthening exercises.

Top 5 Shoulder & Elbow Correction Exercises

1 **All-Fours Rocking Stretch** passively restores normal mechanics of the shoulder and arms.

2 **Wall Slides** teaches proper overhead shoulder mechanics and strengthens the trapezius muscle.

3 **Trapezius Strengthening** strengthens key muscles that control scapular elevation and rotation.

4 **Side-Lying Arm Slides** restores rotator cuff and trapezius strength while improving range of motion.

5 **Assisted Forearm Rotation Stretching** restores range of motion to forearm rotators that contribute to elbow pain.

ALL-FOURS ROCKING STRETCH

This exercise passively restores normal shoulder-joint mechanics. It is a deceptively simple yet powerful exercise that yields big results.

THE FIXING YOU METHOD

Begin in a hands-and-knees position with your hands under your shoulders and knees under your hips. Be sure your lower back is flat by drawing your belly button in toward your spine. Exhale and rock back onto your feet. Feel that the floor is pulling your arms into an overhead position. Allow your shoulders to be pulled into elevation while rocking backward. Essentially the shoulders will shrug up to your ears. Visualize that your scapulae are rotating out without sliding out too far from the spine. Be sure the back of your neck, especially at the base of the skull, remains lengthened.

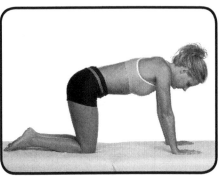

All-Fours Rocking Stretch,
start position

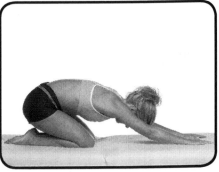

All-Fours Rocking Stretch,
end position

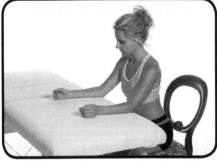

Alternative All-Fours Rocking Stretch,
start position

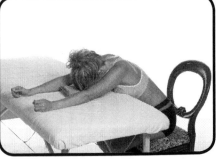

Alternative All-Fours Rocking Stretch,
end position

Feel a nice stretch through your scapula or armpit area. Return to starting position after holding at the bottom for 5 breaths. Perform 3–5 repetitions.

COMMON ERRORS

• Don't round your upper back (thoracic spine) in order to flatten your lower back or to help your arms move into an overhead position. Instead, keep your thoracic spine relaxed and flat.

• Don't let your head to remain up (extended) as you rock down to your feet. Allow your head to slightly flex to your chest, keeping your neck lengthened at the base of your skull.

• You may experience shoulder pain if you try to rock back too far. Stop when you feel any pain.

• Shoulder pain may be caused by rotating your elbow out too far, which impinges the shoulder joint. Try to maintain a neutral elbow, and stop if you feel pain in your shoulder or you can't maintain your arm's neutral position. Keep your elbow creases slightly pointed forward instead of allowing them to rotate inward.

• Maintain adequate elevation of your shoulders. Shrug your shoulders up when you initiate the rocking-back movement; or slide your hands forward prior to rocking back to help pull your shoulders up toward your ears.

WALL SLIDES

This exercise restores normal biomechanics and strengthens key muscles involved in rotating, elevating, and stabilizing the scapulae. I've broken it down into a biomechanics phase and a strengthening phase. Begin strengthening only after you have mastered the biomechanics.

THE FIXING YOU METHOD—BIOMECHANICS

Stand a few inches from the wall so you can comfortably place your elbows and the pinky sides of your hands on the wall as shown. Slide your hands up the wall, making a V shape. When your elbows are level with your shoulders, gradually shrug your shoulders up to help elevate your scapulae. Visualize your scapulae rotating under your arms as they rise and actually helping your arms slide up the wall. Stop before any pain and hold for 5 breaths. Slide your arms down while continuing to shrug your shoulders up. This activates your upper trapezius muscle that has become lengthened or weak. Your arms should be able to fully slide up the wall with elevated scapulae and be pain free. Perform 3–5 repetitions.

COMMON ERRORS

• If your elbows rotate out too much, you may experience shoulder pain. Don't allow the creases of your elbows to rotate into the wall. Keep them facing each other and in the line of the V-shape.

• If you still experience pain in your shoulders, check to make sure that your shoulders are elevating at the right time. Be sure to stop at or prior to pain.

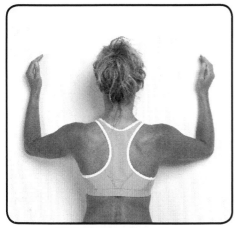
Wall Slides, start position

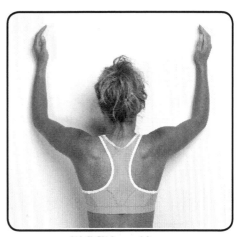
Wall Slides, midway

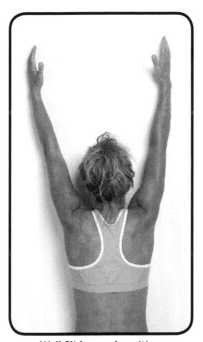
Wall Slides, end position

THE FIXING YOU METHOD—STRENGTHENING

Once your arms are fully elevated and pain free, squeeze your scapulae together to lift your hand off the wall by only 1/4 to 1/2 inch. Be sure to use the scapulae to lift your hands off as opposed to your shoulder muscles.

COMMON ERRORS

•   Not using the scapulae to lift the hands off the wall will cause shoulder pain. As an alternative, perform as a single arm exercise: Reach behind you with your other hand and feel your scapula muscles engage to lift your arm.

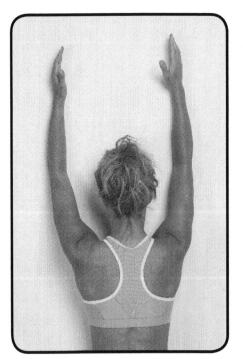

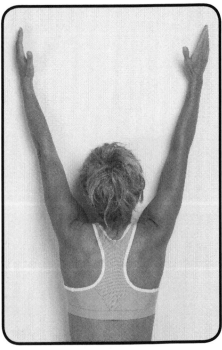

Wall Slides, error
(shoulders have not elevated)

Wall Slides, error
(excessive shoulder internal rotation)

TRAPEZIUS STRENGTHENING

This exercise restores trapezius muscle strength to assist in shoulder elevation and scapular rotation.

THE FIXING YOU METHOD

Lie on your stomach with a pillow or towels under your chest, if necessary, to place less strain on the shoulder and allow greater range of motion to strengthen through. Place your hands on top of your head or neck with elbows resting on the table. Squeeze your scapulae together, then raise your elbows slightly (about 1/4–1/2 inch). Hold for 3–5 breaths, then lower your elbows while maintaining the scapulae contraction. After the elbows are back down to the table, relax the muscles squeezing your scapulae. Perform 5–10 repetitions.

PROGRESSION

Once you can perform this easily, advance by bringing your hands in front of you with elbows bent and thumbs pointed toward the ceiling, similar to a "Superman" position. Now squeeze your scapulae together to raise your arms toward the ceiling.

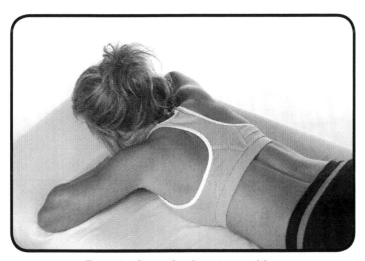

Trapezius Strengthening, start position

COMMON ERRORS

• If you feel pain in your shoulder, be sure your elbow does not rise off the table higher than your wrist. Focus on using your scapulae to raise your elbow rather than using your shoulder joint. Put more pillows under your chest so your arms begin in a more relaxed position.

• If your head arches back, then you can develop neck pain as a result of this exercise. Keep your head down and relaxed. Just focus on the muscles that squeeze the shoulder blades together.

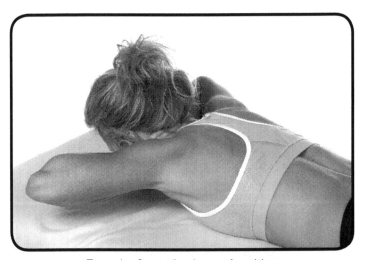

Trapezius Strengthening, end position

ASSISTED FOREARM STRETCH

This exercise restores normal range of motion to the pronators teres and quadratus and supinator muscles of the forearm.

THE FIXING YOU METHOD—FOREARM PRONATION

This requires a friend or physical therapist to help you. While standing, place your shoulders in a biomechanically correct position (scapulae at T2 or T3 and the medial border of the scapula sitting about 3 inches from the spine). Have your friend hold your upper forearm below the elbow and also just above the wrist. They will rotate the hand holding the upper forearm first to rotate your forearm so it is palm down (into pronation). Only rotate your wrist to the point of a nice stretch—not pain. Then ask your friend to gently rotate your wrist into further pronation to accentuate the stretch. Again only rotate the wrist to the point of a nice stretch, not pain. You may not tolerate any more rotation at this point. More is not better. Hold for 30–60 seconds while feeling the stretch. Be sure your shoulders and arm don't move while your forearm is rotated. Give your partner feedback as to whether you are in pain or would like to stretch more. Your partner can increase or decrease the stretch at one or both hands as necessary.

THE FIXING YOU METHOD—FOREARM SUPINATION

Now rotate your forearm so it's palm up (into supination). Have your friend grip your upper forearm and wrist just as above. He or she will rotate your forearm into further supination first using the hand closest to the elbow. Once you feel a nice stretch, then rotate the wrist hand as well. Again stop at the point of a nice stretch—not pain. Hold for 30–60 seconds. Perform 2 repetitions per side, alternating between pronation and supination.

COMMON ERRORS

• Twisting the wrist or upper forearm portion of the forearm too aggressively can cause pain.

• Holding the wrist portion too close to the hand can cause pain.

• Squeezing the forearm too tightly while rotating causes pain.

• Allowing the shoulder to lose its ideal position reduces the stretch.

• The upper arm often will slide out or in during the stretches. In order to get the maximum stretch, don't let it move.

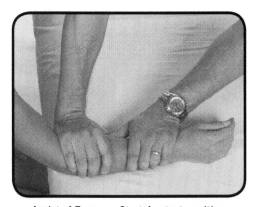

Assisted Forearm Stretch, start position

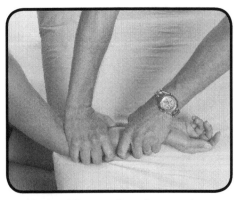

Assisted Forearm Stretch, pronation

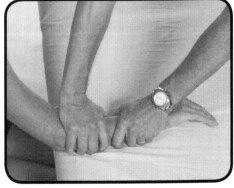

Assisted Forearm Stretch, supination

SHOULDER INTERNAL ROTATOR STRETCH

This exercise helps stretch the teres major, an internal rotator of the arm that runs from the scapula to the humerus. This muscle often becomes excessively tight in people with shoulder or elbow pain.

THE FIXING YOU METHOD

Lie comfortably on your back close to the right edge of a table or bed. Keep your lower back flat on the table. Reach back with your right hand, with elbow bent, to the top of table as shown in the picture below. With your left hand, pull the right elbow toward your head, feeling a stretch in your shoulder blade or arm. Hold for 30–60 seconds and relax. Perform 2–3 repetitions.

COMMON ERRORS

• Pulling too far toward your head will cause shoulder pain.

• Reaching too far back with your right hand may be difficult. If you find that it's too uncomfortable, decrease this range.

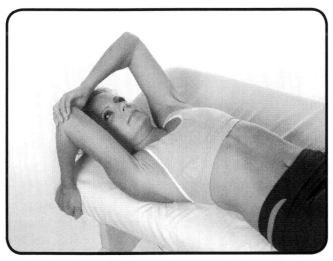

Shoulder Internal Rotator Stretch

ARM WAVES

This exercise helps restore normal range of motion to the shoulder joint and is therefore a powerful tool in fixing shoulder issues. By restoring normal range of motion to the shoulder joint, your arm movements will work independently of your scapulae and diminish the scapulae's influence on elbow dynamics. Internal range of motion should be approximately 70 degrees (fingers touching the table) and external range of motion should be approximately 90 degrees (arm resting on table).

THE FIXING YOU METHOD—INTERNAL ROTATION

Lie on your back with knees supported or bent. Be sure your lower back is comfortable. Rest your right arm on the table in 90 degrees of shoulder abduction as shown below. If your shoulder pops up (possibly due to a tight chest muscle) then support your right arm on a pillow at the elbow to allow the humeral head to more easily sink down toward the table. Place your left hand on your right shoulder to monitor the shoulder joint. It should not pop up during the exercise. Slowly allow your right hand to drift forward and down toward the table. Keep your right shoulder down. Stop if it rises up into your monitoring hand. Allow your right hand to rest in the down position, stretching tight shoulder muscles, for about 30–60 seconds; then return to the starting position, keeping your shoulder down. Repeat while visualizing the muscles in the back or top of your shoulder lengthening to allow your right hand to drift down to the table.

COMMON ERRORS

• If your shoulder pops up immediately when moving your arm, increase the thickness of the padding under your elbow until you can comfortably perform the exercise and feel a stretch. Or decrease the angle of shoulder abduction from 90 degrees to 70 or 60 degrees— whatever allows your shoulder to stay down. As you improve, slide your arm back to a 90-degree position.

• If you feel pain in your shoulder when moving your arm, then you may be trying too hard to push your hand down. Relax and let gravity help you instead.

THE FIXING YOU METHOD—INTERNAL ROTATION
MODIFIED TO SIDE-LYING

This is a good alternative if your shoulders are very tight and you cannot get adequate leverage when lying on your back. Lie down on your right side with your right arm on the floor resting 90 degrees from your body and your elbow bent at 90 degrees so your hand points up toward the ceiling. With your left hand, slowly and gently help your right hand rotate forward, down to the floor. Stop

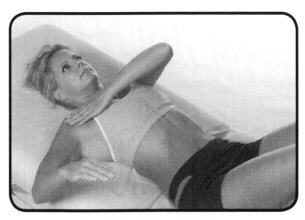

Arm Waves, internal rotation

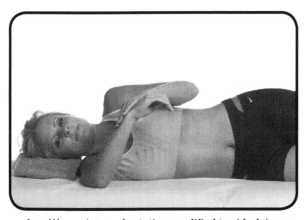

Arm Waves, internal rotation modified to side-lying

once you feel the stretch in the back of your shoulder. Hold for 30–60 seconds and return to the starting position.

THE FIXING YOU METHOD—EXTERNAL ROTATION

This is usually not as difficult for most people. If it isn't difficult for you, then just focus on the internal rotation. While lying on your back with arm out to the side (as in internal rotation), allow your hand to drift back toward your head this time. The shoulder typically won't rise up in this direction, so you need not monitor it. Stop if you feel pain; back off the stretch just enough to avoid the pain.

COMMON ERRORS

• If you experience pain in your shoulder, place thicker pads under your arm until you can feel a stretch with no shoulder pain. Support your wrist and hand with pillows to allow the muscles to relax into the stretch. Otherwise, your shoulder muscles will continue to hold on while trying to stretch and add to joint compression. Slide your elbow down from the 90-degrees abduction position to your side and try again. After the shoulder loosens up, gradually move back into 90 degrees of abduction.

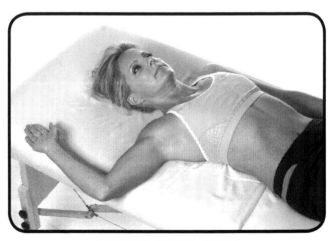

Arm Waves, external rotation

ARM ACROSS CHEST STRETCH

This stretch is very effective for eliminating chronic shoulder pain. It is designed to restore range of motion to the muscles running from the shoulder blade to the arm bone. When these muscles are tight, they contribute to abnormal scapular mechanics.

THE FIXING YOU METHOD—STANDING

Turn sideways to the wall and lean your right shoulder against it. In particular, try to rest the back of your shoulder against the wall; this isolates the scapula so that it cannot slide forward while performing the stretch. Next, with your left hand, grasp your right elbow and pull it across your chest, keeping your right arm low. Feel a stretch without pain. The goal is to eventually get your right elbow to cross the midline of your chest. Hold for 30–60 seconds, then relax and repeat. Perform 3–5 repetitions.

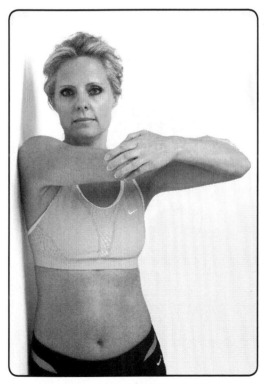

Arm Across Chest Stretch, standing

PROGRESSION

To progress the stretch, elevate your right arm to pull it across your chest at a higher point. Once you can stretch in this range without pain, progress until your arm is approximately shoulder height and pull across your chest.

THE FIXING YOU METHOD—SIDE-LYING

Lie on your right side with your right elbow slightly in front of your trunk. Try to trap your scapula behind you rather than allow it to slide forward underneath you. If you have really tight shoulders, you may have to begin with your elbow closer to your waist. With your left hand, grasp your right elbow and pull it up off the table, toward the ceiling. Feel the stretch in the back or top of your shoulder. Hold for 30–60 seconds, then relax and repeat. Perform 3–5 repetitions. Progress as above by gradually raising your right arm to stretch it across the top of your chest.

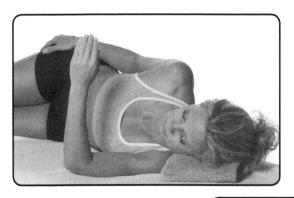

Arm Across Chest Stretch,
side-lying start position

Arm Across Chest Stretch,
side-lying end position

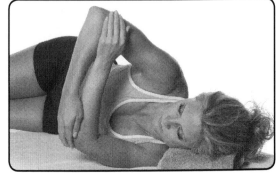

SIDE-LYING ARM SLIDES

This exercise is a real workhorse and restores normal range of motion to the shoulder while strengthening key scapular and rotator cuff muscles. Again, I've broken this down into a biomechanics part and strengthening part. Please begin strengthening only after you have mastered the biomechanics. Range of motion only needs to reach 110–120 degrees of **flexion**.

THE FIXING YOU METHOD—BIOMECHANICS

Lie on your side and rest your top arm on pillows. Be sure your scapula is sitting 3 inches from the spine when beginning and upon returning to the start position. With your thumb pointed toward the ceiling, slide your hand and elbow along the pillow into an overhead position of approximately 110–120 degrees; make sure your elbow does not elevate off the pillow more than your wrist. When your elbow reaches the shoulder level, shrug your shoulder toward your ear to emulate normal overhead biomechanics. Be sure to keep your wrist at the same height or slightly higher than your elbow. Continue sliding your arm up a little higher, maintaining your shrugged shoulder and proper wrist elevation. Hold the position for 5 breaths and return. Perform 2–5 repetitions.

COMMON ERRORS

• If you feel pain in your shoulder, be sure your elbow doesn't rise off the pillow higher than your wrist. Keep your arm heavy on the pillow as you slide it up into a pain-free overhead position. Only slide your arm in a pain-free range of motion.

THE FIXING YOU METHOD—STRENGTHENING

Once in the overhead position, squeeze your scapula to your spine to lift your arm from the pillow. Your arm doesn't need to lift completely off the pillow—just keep its weight off the pillow. Be sure your elbow doesn't rise above your wrist. Hold for 5 breaths. Relax your arm back into the pillow by allowing your scapula to lower it. Slide your arm back down to the starting position and repeat. Perform 3–5 repetitions.

Common Errors

•   If you feel pain in your shoulder, your elbow may have risen higher than your wrist. Also, remember to use your scapular muscles to lift your arm, rather than your shoulder muscles.

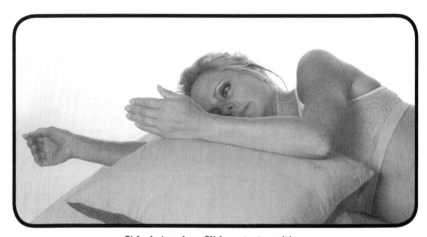

Side-Lying Arm Slides, start position

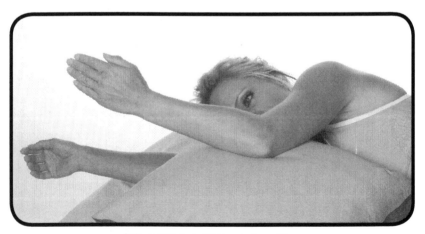

Side-Lying Arm Slides, end position

LATISSIMUS DORSI STRETCH

This exercise restores the latissimus dorsi to its normal length. This muscle originates in the lower back and inserts into the upper arm. When tight, it can alter mechanics of the back, arm, and scapula. Normal shoulder range of motion is 170–180 degrees of flexion. Your arm should basically be able to rest on the table above your head. Your shoulder blade should only slide out approximately 1/2 inch from your trunk. If you experience more abduction than this, have someone block your scapula or try to perform the exercise while controlling this scapular abduction.

THE FIXING YOU METHOD

Lie on your back with knees bent so your lower back remains flat; this anchors one end of the latissimus so you can achieve a better stretch. Draw your belly button in toward your spine to keep your back flat on the ground. Raise your arms overhead by leading with your thumbs as in the picture. Remember the shoulder blades should slide up toward your ears a little as you do this. Feel the stretch in your armpit, ribs, lower back, or upper arm. Make sure

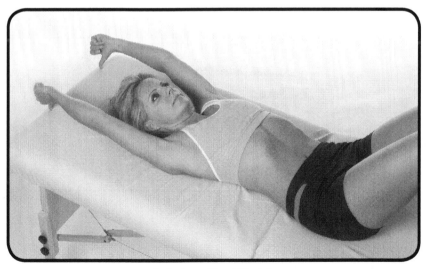

Latissimus Dorsi Stretch

your lower back remains flat throughout the stretch as this is anchoring one end of the latissimus muscle. Hold for 5 breaths or longer. Perform 3–5 repetitions.

COMMON ERRORS

•   If you feel pain in the top of your shoulder, begin the exercise again and stop when you feel a stretch but before pain. Position your arm slightly away from your head. Supporting your arm on a pillow while stretching also helps. Your elbow may have rotated out too far, so monitor it and don't let it rotate.

CHEST STRETCH

This exercise stretches the pectoralis major, which originates from the clavicle (collarbone), sternum, and ribs to attach to the inner part of the upper arm. You should be able to rest your arm at 90–120 degrees of abduction and external rotation as shown.

THE FIXING YOU METHOD

Lie on your back with knees bent to flatten your lower back. Bring your arms out to the side at 90 degrees, as shown. Hold for 30–60 seconds. Be sure your lower back does not arch. Relax, then repeat. Slide the arms up to 120 degrees and stretch there as well. Perform 3–5 repetitions.

COMMON ERRORS

• If you feel pain in your shoulder, place pillows or towels under your arm or wrist to decrease strain on the muscle.

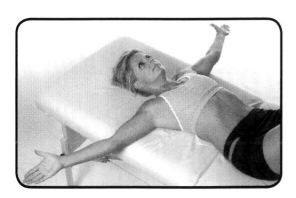

Chest Stretch, 120 degrees

Chest Stretch, 90 degrees

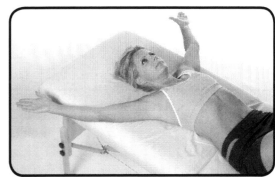

PRONE ARM WAVES

This exercise strengthens the rotator cuff and helps set the humerus correctly in the shoulder socket. It's ideal for correcting an anterior gliding humeral head. Of all the exercises, this is the one that's most difficult for people to feel because many are unaware of how their scapulae are moving. It's best to have someone check this out initially until you can dial it in. Range of motion should be similar to that of Arm Waves.

THE FIXING YOU METHOD

Lie on your stomach with a pillow supporting your left shoulder joint and arm. Be sure your shoulder is not "dropping" down to the table but is instead supported and in line with the scapula. Your lower arm should hang off the edge of the table or rest on towels or pillows to maintain good alignment with the shoul-

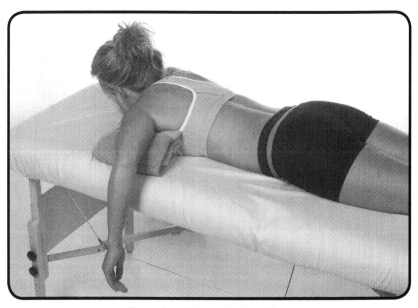

Prone Arm Waves, start position

der. Place your right hand under your left shoulder joint to monitor whether the humeral head is pressing into your hand when performing the exercise. Rotate your left hand up into external rotation without moving the scapula and without allowing the humeral head to push down into your monitoring hand. Don't lift your arm off the pillows but instead maintain constant, steady pressure. Stop if the shoulder presses down into your monitoring hand. Hold for 5 breaths. Slowly return to the starting position, and repeat in the opposite direction. Again, stop if the shoulder presses down into your monitoring hand. Perform 3–5 repetitions.

When performing this exercise in the opposite direction (internal rotation) it will be more difficult to prevent the shoulder from pressing down into your monitoring hand. Be patient and visualize the muscles in the back of your shoulder pulling it up into

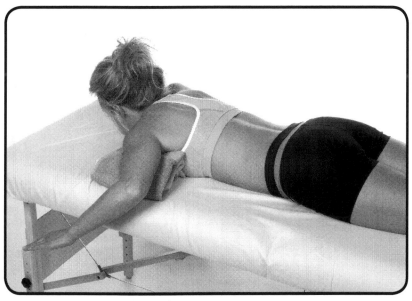

Prone Arm Waves, external rotation

the shoulder socket to prevent the anterior glide. Also be sure not to allow your arm to rise up off the towels or table while moving into internal rotation.

Common Errors

• You may be unable to move your arm without moving your scapula. Be sure you have enough padding under your arm so that the arm bone is in line with your scapula. Begin with small movements, and stop if your scapula moves. Gradually build from there.

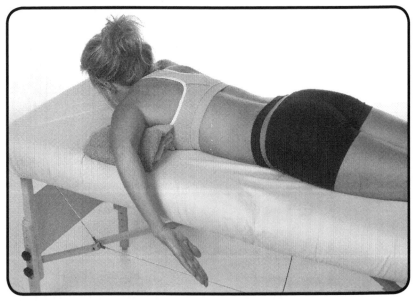

Prone Arm Waves, internal rotation

HAND ON HEAD

This exercise activates the upper trapezius, elevates the shoulder blade, and helps teach you to use your shoulder blade when reaching up with your arm. You can do it almost anywhere.

THE FIXING YOU METHOD

Simply place your hand on top of your head by shrugging your shoulder a little. Relax your arm while maintaining your shrugged shoulder. Be sure your head is in good alignment, not moving forward or cocked to the side. Let the weight of your arm rest on your head.

COMMON ERRORS

•   If you feel pain in your shoulder, try rotating your elbow forward. If this still hurts, then perhaps you don't have adequate range of motion yet. Continue to work on the other exercises.

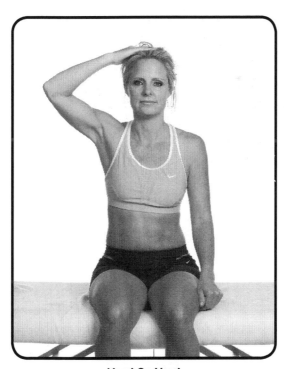

Hand On Head

BICEPS STRETCH

This exercise stretches tight biceps muscles. One of the biceps muscles attaches to the scapula and another to the head of the arm bone. If tight, both muscles can affect shoulder movements by tipping the head of the humerus or scapula forward, which alters shoulder and arm function.

THE FIXING YOU METHOD

Lie on your back with elbow extended and rotate your forearm so the palm of your hand points down and away from you (pronated). Be sure your shoulder doesn't elevate from the table. Slightly rotate your arm to find the best stretch.

COMMON ERRORS

• Stretching too aggressively will cause elbow pain. Place another pillow under your shoulder to decrease the stretch to the biceps and therefore elbow compression.

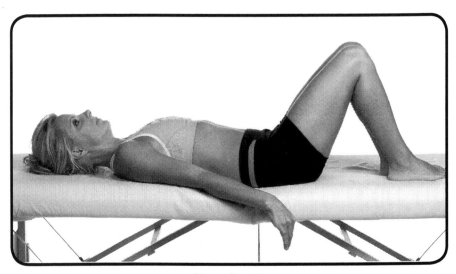

Biceps Stretch

FOREARM ROTATIONAL STRETCHING

This exercise lengthens the pronators teres and quadratus and the supinator muscles of the forearm, which typically cause elbow pain when tight. This exercise is advanced because it requires you to have good control over the rotation of your forearm. The forearm rotator muscles aren't large muscles, so a little weight will go far. I recommend that you stay with the assisted version (page 89) until forearm pain is reduced.

THE FIXING YOU METHOD

Place your shoulders in a biomechanically correct position (scapula at T2 and 3 inches from the spine). Hold a small weight (2–5 pounds) in one hand, as shown. Be sure your shoulder is stable

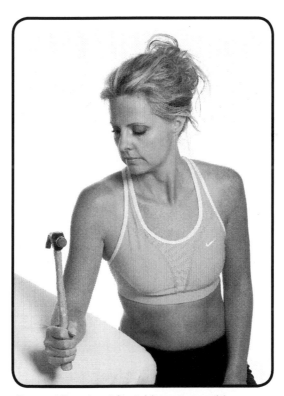

Forearm Rotational Stretching, start position

and does not move during the exercise. Slowly rotate within the fullest range possible without experiencing pain. Visualize your forearm rotating instead of your hand and wrist twisting. Keep your hand at the same angle of rotation as the forearm. You may feel a stretch at the end. Hold the stretch for 15–30 seconds. Don't allow your upper arm bone to rotate; we only want the forearm to rotate. Stop at the end range of motion or if it is painful. Rotate into the opposite direction and maintain a pain-free stretch for 15–30 seconds. You can also try this while standing, similar to the assisted version. Perform 3–5 repetitions.

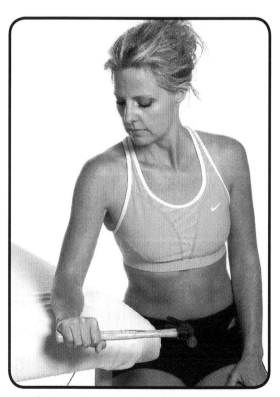

Forearm Rotational Stretching, pronation

COMMON ERRORS

• If the upper arm bone (humerus) and/or shoulder move, the weights will rotate more than they should.

• Don't rotate the weights too quickly.

• Don't allow your wrist and hand to twist instead of your forearm.

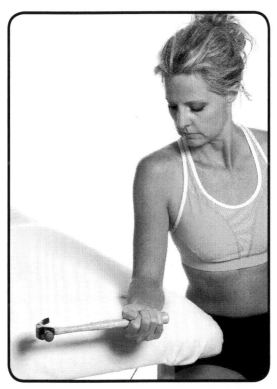

Forearm Rotational Stretching, supination

ASSISTED FOREARM ROTATION STRENGTHENING

This exercise restores normal range of motion and strength to the pronator and supinator muscles of the forearm. It's important to restore proper strength to the rotator muscles through the entire range of motion, especially for people who work with their hands or athletes such as golfers. This will help prevent a recurrence of elbow pain.

THE FIXING YOU METHOD

This exercise requires a friend or therapist to help you. Place your shoulders in a biomechanically correct position. Hold your elbow at a 90-degree angle at your side while holding a dowel rod or broom handle in your hand. Have your partner slowly turn the rod while you gently resist and allow your forearm to rotate until the full range of motion is achieved or you feel pain. Feel your forearm muscles resisting the rotation and your shoulder blade muscles working to hold your shoulder blade in the correct position. This should take about 15–30 seconds to perform one rotation. Reverse the direction and repeat. Perform 3–5 repetitions or until fatigue sets in.

COMMON ERRORS
- Twisting the rod too quickly can cause pain.
- Resisting with too much force can cause pain.
- Rotating too far can cause pain.

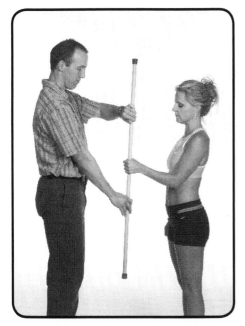

Assisted Forearm Rotation Strengthening,
start position

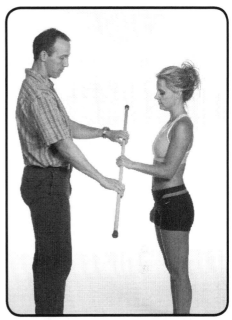

Assisted Forearm Rotation Strengthening,
moving into pronation

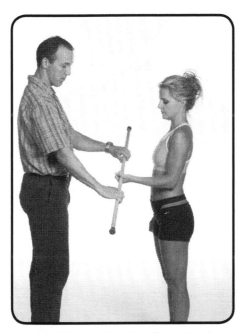

Assisted Forearm Rotation Strengthening,
moving into supination

Conclusion

I hope you've gained an appreciation for the fact that the shoulder is a one-of-a-kind joint in the body. This ball-and-socket joint has unparalleled freedom of movement. What makes it especially unique is that its base of support, the scapula, also moves. This allows for a variety of movements and functions of the arm and hand as evidenced by an almost unlimited spectrum of sports and work environments the shoulder must both adapt to and excel at.

The scapula's position on the trunk helps determine how well the arm bone moves in its socket. Muscles also play a role here, specifically the latissimus dorsi and pectoralis muscles. These large muscle groups can overwhelm small rotator cuff muscles, creating an environment for shoulder pain.

You've also learned how the scapula affects elbow pain. I don't believe any of the clients' elbow pain I helped would have been able to heal had it not been for addressing the shoulder blade as well. Again, the chest and back muscles also come into play here. By excessively internally rotating the arm bone, they create a poor environment in which the forearm muscles must work.

But learning about all of these mechanics is only half the battle. Now you must practice the exercises and fix yourself. Each exercise has a role to play in eliminating your shoulder and elbow pain. In a fast-paced world, it's difficult to take time to really absorb information, but I hope you have.

In my experience, those who really "get into it" are rewarded the most in the form of rapid pain reduction, improved performance, and injury prevention. You now have the knowledge to fix your injuries—you only need to apply it. It often requires very little intervention before experiencing significant pain reduction. I wish you luck on your road to self-discovery and improved human performance!

FIXING YOU: SHOULDER & ELBOW PAIN

GLOSSARY

abducting
Moving away from the midline of the body out to the side. For example, when moving an arm out to the side, the arm is abducting.

abduction
A position that results from abducting an appendage. For example, an arm held out to the side is said to be in abduction.

acromion—See scapula.

adducting
Moving toward the body. For example, the process of bringing the arm back to the side of the body from abduction is said to be adducting the arm.

adduction
The position of an appendage closer to the body relative to abduction.

anterior
In front or forward; the opposite of posterior. For instance, anterior pelvic tilt occurs when the top of the pelvis is tilted forward.

anterior glide
When a bone in a joint slides forward in a socket more than it should normally slide.

anterior tilt
A scapula that is rotated forward is said to be anteriorly tilted. Often a scapula that is anteriorly tilted, is unable to posteriorly tilt during arm raising.

biceps (biceps brachii)
An upper arm muscle composed of two heads, a long head and a short head. This muscle flexes the elbow and shoulder as well as supinates the forearm.

> **long head:** Originates just above the shoulder socket on the scapula and blends with the short head on to the radius bone of the forearm.

> **short head:** Originates on the coracoid process of the scapula and blends with the long head on to the radius bone of the forearm.

bursitis
Inflammation of a fluid-filled sac (bursa), which lies between a tendon and skin or tendon and bone.

cervical vertebrae
Seven vertebrae compose the neck portion of the spine. The cervical vertebrae naturally have a degree of lordotic curve also found in the lumbar spine.

clavicle
Collar bone which attaches to the trunk at the sternum and the shoulder at the AC joint.

coracoid process—See scapula.

deltoid muscle
The shoulder muscle originating from the clavicle and scapula and inserting onto the lateral portion of the humerus. The front (anterior) fibers help flex the arm, lateral fibers help abduct the arm and back (posterior) fibers help extend the arm.

depressed scapula
A scapula that is resting lower on the trunk than it should.

epicondyles
The bony ridges on either side of the humerus near the elbow joint.

epicondylitis
Inflammation of an epicondyle.

extending
The act of straightening a joint or reversing a flexed position. Extending an elbow involves straightening the elbow joint.

extension
Describes a position relative to a neutral or flexed position.

external rotation
Also referred to as lateral rotation. Rotating the anterior surface of a bone or joint away from the midline of the body.

external rotators (shoulders)
Muscles attaching to the scapula that externally rotate the arm.

infraspinatus: Originates on the vertebral border of the scapula and inserts onto the humerus.

teres minor: Smaller than the infraspinatus, it originates on the vertebral border of the scapula and inserts onto the humerus.

supraspinatus: Originates above the spine of the scapula and inserts into the humeral head.

flexing
The act of bending a joint.

flexion
Describes a position that is flexed relative to neutral or extension. An elbow is in flexion when it is bent. A spine is in flexion when it is bent forward.

functional problem
When the body does not move correctly due to weakness, impaired range of motion, previous injury, or habitual movement patterns. Functional problems typically create pain and may cause physical changes to tissues.

golfer's elbow—See medial epicondylitis.

humerus
The upper arm bone. The head of the humerus interacts with the socket of the scapula to form the shoulder joint.

hyperextended
A joint that extends too far or too easily is said to be hyperextended.

hypermobile
A joint that has too much motion, which may or may not be well controlled. A hypermobile joint often occurs near a hypomobile joint.

hypomobile
A joint that has too little motion. When a joint does not move well, other joints above or below it typically must compensate by becoming hypermobile in order to achieve functional movement.

impingement
Pinched or compressed tissue, usually between two bones or mus-

cles. For instance, a nerve may become impinged if it is pinched between two vertebrae.

inferior angle—See scapula.

infraspinatus—See external rotators.

internal rotation
Rotating the anterior surface of a bone or joint toward the midline of the body; also referred to as medial rotation. For instance, rotating a knee inward so that it points toward the midline of the body is internally rotating the knee.

internal rotators (shoulder)
Muscles attaching to the humerus that internally rotate the arm.

> **latissimus dorsi:** Originates on the lower thoracic and lumbar vertebrae as well as iliac crest. It attaches to the inferior angle of the scapula as it travels up to insert on the humerus. Along with contributing to excessive internal rotation of the arm or scapular abduction, the latissimus dorsi also contributes to extension problems when tight or when the abdominals are weak.

> **pectoralis major:** Originates along the clavicle, down the sternum, and across the ribs and inserts into the humerus. This muscle can contribute to excessive internal rotation of the arm or scapular abduction.

> **teres major:** Originates on the scapula and inserts onto the humerus. When tight, this muscle contributes to scapular abduction and excessive internal rotation of the arm.

> **subscapularis:** Originates on the underside of the scapula and inserts onto the humerus. When tight, this muscle contributes to scapular abduction and excessive internal rotation of the arm.

joint capsule
A dense, fibrous connective tissue surrounds our joints providing stability and assisting with coordinating movement.

labrum
Both the shoulder and hip sockets have a ring of thick cartilage around them which deepens the socket and provides stability for

the humeral or femoral heads as they move in the socket.

lateral epicondylitis
Inflammation of the outer (lateral) epicondyle of the humerus; also called tennis elbow.

latissimus dorsi—See internal rotators.

levator scapula
Originates at the scapula and inserts into the first four cervical vertebrae. Can contribute to excessive movements of the cervical spine.

Medial epicondylitis
Inflammation of the inner (medial) epicondyle of the humerus; also called golfer's elbow.

movement dysfunction
A way of moving that is unnatural to optimal biomechanics and can cause pain; also referred to as movement fault.

pectoralis major—See internal rotators.

pectoralis minor
A deep chest muscle originating at ribs 3–5 and inserting into the corocoid process of the scapula. When tight, this muscle can pull the scapula forward altering its axis of rotation.

posterior
Behind or in back of; the opposite of anterior. For instance, posterior pelvic tilt occurs when the top of the pelvis is tilted backward.

posterior tilt
The movement of the scapula to rotate down and back during arm raising. This allows the supraspinatus muscle to function unimpinged.

pronation
A rotational movement typically associated with the forearm and hand as well as the foot. Regarding the hand, this involves rotating it palm down.

pronator muscles (forearm)
Muscles that pronate the forearm. When tight, these muscles may contribute to tennis and golfer's elbow.

Pronator quadratus: Located near the wrist this muscle connects the radius and ulna.

Pronator teres: Originates on the medial side of the humerus and inserts into the radius.

prone
Term given to the body position in which a person is lying on his or her stomach.

radius
One of the forearm bones.

rhomboid
Muscles that originate at the mid-thoracic spine and attach to the vertebral border of the scapula. They are important for scapular positioning and movement.

rotator cuff
Term given to the shoulder muscles running from the scapula to the arm bone. (See internal rotators and external rotators for more detail.)

scapula
Also known as the shoulder blade. This bone articulates with the humerus to form the shoulder joint. Scapular function is important to preventing or fixing shoulder and neck injuries. It is shaped in a triangle.

vertebral border: The border which is closest and runs roughly parallel to the spine.

coracoid process: Protrudes anteriorly and to which the pectoralis minor attaches.

acromion: A bony lip of the scapula that forms the "roof" of the shoulder joint. The acromion and clavicle come together (articulate) to form the AC joint (acromioclavicular joint).

inferior angle: The bottom corner of the scapula.

spine: A ridge along the scapula that terminates in the acromion. The infraspinatus, teres major, and teres minor originate below the spine, and the supraspinatus originates above the spine. The spine is palpated to assess scapular position on the trunk.

serratus anterior
This muscle originates on the front, or lateral, ribs and inserts onto the vertebral border of the scapula. It is important for scapular positioning and movement.

structural diagnosis
A diagnosis describing a physical change in the body such as a bulging disk or arthritis.

subacromial space
The space between the acromion of the scapula and the head of the humerus in which the supraspinatus muscle works. Impingement of this muscle is common due to narrowing of the subacromial space.

subscapularis—See internal rotator muscles.

supination
A rotational movement typically associated with the forearm and hand as well as the foot. Regarding the hand, this involves rotating it to face palm up.

supinator
A forearm muscle responsible for supinating the forearm and hand. It originates at the lateral bone of the humerus and inserts into the radius.

supine
Term given to the body position in which a person is lying on his or her back.

supraspinatus muscle—See external rotators.

tennis elbow—See lateral epicondylitis.

teres major—See internal rotators.

teres minor—See external rotators.

thoracic vertebra—See vertebrae.

trapezius
A large muscle group of the shoulder, neck and upper back. The trapezius muscle is important to shoulder function and is divided into three zones.

> **upper:** Originates at the base of the skull and down a thick ligament connecting to the spine. It inserts into the clavicle and acromion process of the scapula. This portion elevates the scapula during arm movements, stabilizes the scapula during adduction, and assists with rotation.

> **mid:** Originates from vertebrae 1–5 and inserts into the acromion and spine of the scapula. This portion adducts and stabilizes during scapular rotation.

> **lower:** Originates from vertebrae 6–12 and inserts into the spine of the scapula. This portion depresses and rotates the scapula.

triceps
Posterior muscles of the upper arm that extend the shoulder and the elbow. They are composed of two heads.

> **long head:** Originates at the scapula and inserts along with the lateral and medial heads into the elbow. This muscle assists with shoulder adduction and extension as well as elbow extension.

> **lateral head:** Originates on the outer surface of the humerus. This portion inserts along with the long and medial heads into the elbow.

> **medial head:** Originates on the medial surface of the humerus and inserts along with the lateral and long heads into the elbow.

trigger point
A hypersensitive point or nodule in muscle that, when pressed, can refer pain to a distant site.

ulna
One of the forearm bones that articulates with the humerus.

vertebrae (singular vertebra)
The bones that comprise the spine. They are divided into three sections.

> **cervical:** The neck region. There are seven cervical vertebrae. They form an inward lordotic curve.

> **thoracic:** The upper trunk region where ribs attach. There are twelve thoracic vertebrae. They form an outward kyphotic curve.

> **lumbar:** The lower spine region composed of five vertebrae. They form an inward lordotic curve.

vertebral border—See scapula.

About the Author

Rick Olderman MSPT, CPT

Following graduation in 1996 from the nationally ranked Krannert School of Physical Therapy at the University of Indianapolis, I practiced at a small sports and orthopedic clinic in Cortez, Colorado. Because the clinic had a small gym attached, I was able to progress patients to a higher functional level than if I were in a typical clinic. This unique model influenced me to consider personal training. I discovered that setting up therapeutic training programs for my patients helped them as much or more than any intervention I would perform manually.

I moved to Denver in 1999 and began working as a physical therapist and personal trainer at an exclusive health club, The Athletic Club at Denver Place. While there, I continued to experiment with blending rehabilitation and personal training and added Pilates to my skill set. Within just a few months, I became the top-producing employee at the club. I held that position for the next four years until I opened my own studio/clinic.

In addition to providing individual client services, I also lead corporate seminars for injury prevention and correction. My focus on teaching employees the fundamentals of injury mechanics and practical ways to correct them has made me an effective force in changing corporate thinking about injuries, injury prevention, ergonomics, and fitness programs. I believe education is the key. I find that if you teach someone how the body works and why they experience pain, most people will be more diligent in helping themselves. No one wants to be in pain.

I am an active member of the American Physical Therapy Association, and I continue to explore combined rehabilitation and fitness techniques through professional development and continuing education. I live and work in Denver, Colorado with my wife and two young children.

REFERENCES

Introduction opening quote:
Nechis, Barbara. 1993. *Watercolor from the Heart*. New York: Watson-Guptill Publications.

Section 1 opening quote:
Yogananda, Paramahansa. 1997. *Journey to Self-Realization*. Los Angeles, CA: Self-Realization Fellowship.

Section 2 opening quote:
Chopra, Deepak. 1993. *Creating Affluence: Wealth Consciousness in the Field of All Possibilities*. San Rafael, CA: New World Library.

Section 3 opening quote:
Campbell, Joseph. 1991. *The Joseph Campbell Companion: Reflections on the Art of Living*. Ed. Diane K. Osbon. New York: HarperCollins.

Kendall, Florence, Elizabeth McCreary, and Patricia Provance. 1993. *Muscles: Testing and Function, with Posture and Pain*. Fourth edition. Baltimore, MD: Williams & Wilkins.

Sahrmann, Shirley A. 2002. *Diagnosis and Treatment of Movement Impairment Syndromes*. St. Louis, MO: Mosby.

To access your free video demonstrations of all exercises in this book, visit **www.FixingYou.net**, select the Shoulder & Elbow Pain book under the "Books" tab at the top, and then click the "View Video Clips" button. Once on the video clip page, type in the code: **latissimus**.

Printed in Great Britain
by Amazon.co.uk, Ltd.,
Marston Gate.